Hospital Babylon

www.**rbooks**.co.uk

Hospital Babylon

IMOGEN EDWARDS-JONES
& Anonymous

BANTAM PRESS

LONDON • TORONTO • SYDNEY • AUCKLAND • JOHANNESBURG

TRANSWORLD PUBLISHERS
61–63 Uxbridge Road, London W5 5SA
A Random House Group Company
www.rbooks.co.uk

First published in Great Britain
in 2011 by Bantam Press
an imprint of Transworld Publishers

This book is a fictional account based on the experiences and recollections
of the author's sources. In some cases, names and sequences or the detail
of events have been changed to protect the privacy of others. The author
has stated to the publishers that, except in such respects not
affecting the substantial accuracy of the work, the contents
of this book are true.

A CIP catalogue record for this book
is available from the British Library.

ISBNs 9780593066300 (hb)
9780593066317 (tpb)

Addresses for Random House Group Ltd companies outside the UK
can be found at www.randomhouse.co.uk
The Random House Group Ltd Reg. No. 954009

The Random House Group Limited supports The Forest Stewardship
Council (FSC), the leading international forest-certification organization. All our
titles that are printed on Greenpeace-approved FSC-certified paper carry the FSC logo.
Our paper procurement policy can be found at
www.rbooks.co.uk/environment

Typeset in 11.5/16pt Sabon by
Falcon Oast Graphic Art Ltd.
Printed and bound in Great Britain by
Clays Ltd, Bungay, Suffolk

2 4 6 8 10 9 7 5 3 1

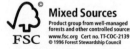

Mixed Sources
Product group from well-managed
forests and other controlled sources
www.fsc.org Cert no. TT-COC-2139
© 1996 Forest Stewardship Council
FSC

For Jane G

With love and thanks
for absolutely everything

Acknowledgements

With very grateful thanks to the extremely talented and highly entertaining doctors, nurses, shrinks, consultants and mid-wives who I interviewed for this book. I am wholly indebted to them for their humour, generosity, trust, patience, hard work, endless explanation, great anecdotage, and most of all their time. I couldn't have done it without them. Thank you also to the wonderful Eugenie Furniss, the handsome Doug Young, the fabulous Laura Sherlock, the dashing Larry Finlay, and all at Transworld for their fabulousness. Nothing would get done, written or indeed published without you. Thank you all.

Prologue

All of the following is true. Only the names have been changed to protect the guilty. All the anecdotes, the situations, the highs, the lows, the drugs, the excesses, the waste, the sadness and the insanity are as told to me by Anonymous – a collection of some of the finest and most successful consultants, doctors, nurses and physicians in the country. The hospital, for legal reasons, is fictionalized, but the incidents and cases are real. Narrated by Anonymous, all these stories have been condensed into a twenty-four-hour time frame. But everything else is as it should be. The drunks vomit, the addicts keel over, babies are born and young men continue to shoot and stab each other – and doctors and nurses clear up the mess.

7–8 a.m.

I am sweating and shaking and feeling really quite nauseous. My head is pounding like some shit seventies disco due to extreme dehydration, and if I didn't know better I'd swear I can actually hear my liver screaming. This isn't good. This is not very clever. Even this bus window my head is currently using for support is making me feel ill. I can barely stomach the smell of the tepid bacon sandwich in my bag, let alone eat it. Christ. I haven't felt this rubbish in years.

Normally I am quite professional when it comes to a hangover. Well, at least I was, in the olden days when I worked an almost hundred-hour weekend – Friday morning till Monday evening – with about two hours' sleep a night. Thursday night was party night, even if I did have to work a solid four days afterwards. It was a matter of pride. We used to down as much vodka as we could and still make it back to the halls of residence, where we'd buddy up with a fellow pissed student doctor and spend the next twenty minutes trying to cannulate each other, sticking IV drips into each other's arms with litre fluid bags attached and then settling back for a big old snooze while we gently rehydrated ourselves, so as to turn up at work the next day bright-eyed, relatively bushy-tailed and totally devoid of hangover. Occasionally this master plan would go tits up, so to speak. If you were one of those restless flailing-around-in-the-bed drunks, you had to be careful. My room mate Julian was one, and I lost count of the number of times he kicked the IV stand over and knocked the bag to the ground, lower than his heart, so that instead of hydrating himself he bled into the thing like some unconscious haemophiliac. We'd wake up the next day and it was like there'd been a murder. Bloody blood bloody everywhere. The worst time was when he lost over a litre and ended up having to do a shift hungover, exhausted and completely anaemic.

Not that it made that much of a difference. Both of us were pretty shit on Friday mornings. We used to do cardiology and eventually the poor bastard consultant got rather bored of teaching us – or, more precisely, dragging us kicking and stinking around the ward as we scratched down some notes and smiled vacantly at patients. No one ever answered him when he posed supposedly intellectually fascinating conundrums. It must have been quite frustrating for the old boy. Julian and I would get through the morning somehow and then carbo-load at lunch in the hospital mess, shovelling in as much fish and chips and ketchup as we could get down our gullets, and then we'd go back to the ward ready for action, redoing the notes and consultations we were supposed to have done before lunch. The only evidence that we had been there before was traces of our scrawled handwriting. We would, of course, have no memory of it at all.

But still, sitting here on the bus, I rather wish I had bothered to root around for a vein last night, as I would be feeling a hell of a lot better than I am now. Even my tongue feels thick and spongy and too big for my mouth. The problem is my girlfriend, Emma, doesn't like IVs in the house. She's a civilian. She works in an office and keeps normal hours and has a normal life and doesn't think that self-medicating is OK, or indeed charming, and I haven't been with her for long so I am trying to keep on the straight and narrow so as not to scare her away. Put it this way: she hasn't met Julian yet.

Sadly, I haven't seen him for a while either. He's off doing obstetrics down in some provincial hell hole in the south-west, getting in his requisite number of complicated births, or whatever this week's government guidelines are, before he can move on to something a little more relaxing and a little less on the front line. I can't believe he is now specializing in obstetrics and gynaecology, but then he has always been a bit crazy. It doesn't seem very long ago now that he was donning a crash helmet on the roof of the Royal London, about to run like a bastard towards the edge of the building, hoping to hurl himself over its side, into the helicopter safety nets.

On long hot balmy summer days a gang of us juniors used to gather together to get extremely drunk and have barbecues on top of the hospital. We'd pack a whole load of stuff – beer, bangers and IVs – and head for the roof in the hope that the fire brigade didn't ring the red bat phone downstairs and scramble a chopper and the trauma team for some severe incident or other. Anyway, as the sun went down we'd knock back the beers, burn the sausages and get out the propofol. Otherwise known as 'milk of amnesia', propofol is very fast-acting and is used to knock patients out – some, most famously Michael Jackson, a little bit more profoundly than others. We used to race with it. We'd start in the middle of the helipad, put a helmet on, inject the propofol and then run as fast as we could towards the edge of the building before keeling over. The aim was to sprint as fast as you could and flop over the side into the safety nets, to be hauled out a few minutes later as you came round. Fall short, as I did, and you ended up passing out on the roof and grazing yourself on the helipad. Needless to say, Julian got to the nets every time.

He was also, by all accounts, excellent at the Sux Races at one London hospital. These legendary events take place in a particular ward where the corridors are nice and long. Julian and co. would inject suxamethonium, an incapacitating drug we sometimes use before intubating someone, and then run as fast as they could down the corridor before they became paralysed. The person who managed to sprint the furthest before twitching frantically and becoming completely immobile was, naturally, the winner. Total paralysis, but fully conscious with it – a kind of living hell, really. The dangers of the game are obvious. Although try to tell doctors about drugs and they always think they know best. But, just because we're familiar with their names, components and side effects doesn't actually mean we totally understand them.

That doesn't stop us from helping ourselves, if and when we

fancy it. I have certainly lifted a few bits and bobs, vials and pills, in search of a good time. Nothing too serious, like diamorphine, which is about two grand an ampoule and requires more signatures than the Kyoto Protocol to get your hands on, but some more entertaining things like the odd canister of nitrous oxide, or laughing gas, to get a party going, or a few GTN patches here and there. Glyceryl trinitrate dilates the blood vessels. It's more usually used to treat angina or a heart attack, but pop one on before sex and it makes the whole thing go with much more of a bang, so to speak. So does Cialis. A milder form of Viagra and prescribed for erectile dysfunction, it is so popular at a mate of mine's shrink practice that they usually run out of their Friday delivery of the stuff by lunchtime. It is so regularly pilfered by the doctors and the staff that last week when he prescribed some for a patient he had to go through his partner's desk to get his hands on a packet or two.

I look out of the window. It's my stop. I'd better get a move on. It may be my last day in A&E but I can't be late. I say it's my last day; it is not my last day as a doctor. I have spent the last eight years of my life training to be one so that would be a bit of a waste. It is my last day in this particular Accident and Emergency. I'm doing the eight a.m. to six p.m. shift and then I'm off to another hospital, St Patrick's, up the road, to do a six-month stint in Acute Medicine before I get sent somewhere else again. But this week it's all change. It's all change every-where in the NHS. It's the first Wednesday in August. The day when all the new student doctors, freshly graduated from medical school, take up their posts, and also the day when every doctor all over the country who is still training moves. The consultants and nurses stay, but the rest of us, like some huge rotating carousel, are released back into the community and moved on to pastures new. They always say the first Wednesday in August is the worst day of the year to get ill. You are 6 per cent more likely to die on 'Black Wednesday' than at any other time of year. Wherever you are in the country, whatever NHS department you are in, everyone is new. The newly qualified junior doctors have no idea what they are doing. And the rest of us don't know where the toilets are, let alone how to turn the oxygen on, who's in charge of the morphine, or which is the quickest way to the intensive care unit. It's like some morbid medical double whammy.

But that's tomorrow. We still have today to get through first. And it's raining. It's supposed to be summer. It's so typical. It's not even real rain. It's drizzling. It's grey, it's drizzling, and my head hurts. Still, only one more shift to go and then freedom! Well, perhaps not freedom, but maybe a bit of respect?

A&E is universally acknowledged to be the worst department to work in in the whole hospital, and that includes the renal unit, Geriatrics and Sexually Transmitted Diseases. It is viewed as the worst mainly because it is hard to do a good job. A&E is still about waiting times and getting people in and out as quickly as possible. All you can do is just enough either to patch them up and send them home or move them through the system to somewhere else. When we call up another department asking for tests or a bed, we are usually met with a long litany of sighs and an attitude of general irritation at the idea of yet another hopeless referral from A&E. Outside the charming confines of medicine, people think that Accident and Emergency has a whiff of glamour, a touch of George Clooney about it, with plenty of striding around, some fondling of a stethoscope, and the occasional helping hand given to distressed women giving birth. But inside medicine they look down on us somewhat. The phrase 'Jack of all trades' gets bandied about a lot, and in a world which is all about specializing and where knowing an awful lot about a thyroid is considered very important, being good at lots of things is not something to aspire to.

Walking through the main entrance to the hospital, I nod vaguely at the dozy-looking bloke on main reception. He looks completely through me. I've only been working here for six months, smiling and nodding at him nearly every day, and still my face draws a blank. I'm not sure what it would take to burn any sort of image into his uninspired brain. I pass the newsagent selling crisps, carnations and cheap faded paper-backs, and on up the stairs to A&E.

Through the swing doors, and the air is stultifyingly thick. I never know why hospitals are always so damn hot. They say it's to keep the old and infirm warm, but I always think, much like they turn the temperature up in aircraft when they want the passengers to fall asleep, they use the heat in here to keep the patients docile.

And then the smell hits me. That hospital smell. Sweet and sickly. A heady cocktail of disinfectant, damp clothes, dust, rotting food, stale breath, urine and illness. Normally I can cope with it, but today it makes me retch and my eyes water. I'll be used to it in a minute. What I wouldn't give for two litres of Hartmann's fluids and a 1-gram IV of plain old paracetamol. If I am very very nice to Sister, I wonder, might she actually give me some? Then again, I could always pinch it before my shift starts. Although we had an anaesthetist last week who pinched an anti-emetic called metoclopramide to stop herself from feeling lousy; unfortunately she had a bit of a reaction to it and ended up twitching and convulsing on the floor in front of her own patient. Not a good look. I think perhaps I shall stick to a full fat Coke from the drinks machine instead.

Just along the corridor from the waiting room are the staff changing rooms, divided up into sexes, though we share the old tin lockers and rows of school pegs with the male nurses. The nurses have their own lockers but for some reason the doctors have to share. I suppose they think we won't be here long; either that or they think we don't have anything worth pinching. I have to say that I've learnt to bring nothing into this hospital that I don't mind 'sharing' with others. Everything gets nicked here. I don't know who does it. The doctors? Nurses? Orderlies? Cleaning staff? Patients? Anything that is not nailed down or sewn into your pockets gets lifted. iPhones are a particular favourite so I always try and hide mine – not that I have the time to chat or text. Still, as one sanguine old consultant once said to me when his medical instruments disappeared, 'It is a great measure of how good they are.'

I dump my old jeans and T-shirt in a fortuitously empty locker, hide my iPhone in a hanky in my jeans pocket and leaf through the pile of blue scrubs on the bench to find something resembling my size. They are colour-coded around the neck as well as having a coloured cord hanging off the trousers which announces to the world that you are small, medium, large or extra-large, which is fine if you are a bloke but less fine for some of the girls who have to declare their ever-expanding plumpness to the entire community every time they slip on a white large or a pink extra-large top. We wear scrubs because we are more or less guaranteed to be sprayed in blood, urine or vomit at least once during the shift. The consultants who run the show and are therefore one step away from the general public used to wear suits, or just shirtsleeves – their arms were supposed to be naked from the elbow down for hygiene reasons. These days, however, they have to wear aprons which make them look like senior nurses, or, as one livid bloke put it the other day, 'like we are manning the bloody cheese counter at Tesco'. It is not a popular change, as you can imagine.

But then there are many changes around here that are not at all popular. One of the least popular is the alterations they've made to doctor training. Doctors used to be quite a strong body. We are a bolshie lot, hard to sack and control. However, the way to disempower us is to train too many of us, creating more training posts than there are jobs available, so that we end up in limbo, swilling around in the system, vainly hoping that something will turn up. We get a lot of these limbo doctors in A&E. With no consultancy available to them, they end up working locum shifts here in order to make ends meet.

Although all this is about to change again with the new government's plan. Quite what a huge effect it will have on us is anyone's guess. Some of us are excited, but most are not. Past experience has shown that when it comes to change, the

NHS is about as flexible as an 85-year-old geriatric with gout. There are corridors, wings and whole hospitals that are atrophied with initiatives and good intentions. Most of us expect a huge haemorrhage of cash followed by a mad-dash attempt to resuscitate the beast, while the rest of the medical profession watches on, shaking its head, saying, 'I told you so.' Or it could work!

A short walk down the corridor, I go into the common room to eat my now cold bacon sandwich and get a Coke from the drinks machine. It is not the most salubrious of places with its filthy sofas, biodegrading chairs and ancient botulin-riddled fridge, but it's a place to store your lunch, munch on your crisps, and get the gossip. A clutch of medical posters curl off the wall, alongside lists of pink, blue and green teams for the nurses' rotas, as well as a cork noticeboard filled with handwritten notes about flat shares or lame adverts for yoga, aqua-aerobics or the early signs of diabetes.

'Oh, hello stranger! I can't believe you made it in,' declares a round blonde called Margaret, who is one of the few pretty nurses we have in A&E. She squeezes a Sainsbury's bag in between three Tupperware boxes on the top shelf of the fridge, before turning to look at me.

'Ha ha,' I reply, squinting slightly as I stare into the palm of my hand, looking for the correct change for the drinks machine.

'No, I'm serious,' she says. 'You were last seen dancing to "I'm Every Woman" in a pink Afro wig.'

'Dancing?' I stop what I'm doing. I seriously don't remember the wig or the song or the dance. I don't normally dance. Shit.

I must have been extremely drunk.

My heart is now beating a little fast and I am beginning to sweat.

'Still,' she shrugs, 'at least you weren't discovered in the medical store on all fours giving Mr Mukti a blow job like Lorraine in ICU.'

'Dr Lorraine?' I ask, like it makes a difference.

'No, physio Lorraine,' replies Margaret.

'It's always the physios,' interjects the head nurse, folding her arms, as she queues up behind me to use the drinks machine. Short and dark with a bosom the size of a sofa, Sister Andrea is not the sort of woman you want to mess with, in every sense of the word. 'They are quite the party animals.'

'I must say I didn't see any of your lot holding back when it came to the drinks,' I say, remembering trying to elbow my way through the scrum of nurses who were about two to three deep at the bar.

'Yes, well,' she says, pursing her lips slightly as she looks up my nose. 'At least my girls can dance.'

Making a tit of yourself at the annual mess party is de rigueur, especially if you are leaving the place. Every hospital has a few huge piss-ups a year and the plusher the hospital the posher the piss-up; a few of them, like the Chelsea and Westminster and St Mary's Paddington, even have a couple of black tie or fancy dress balls on top. However, every hospital has a mess that all the doctors and nurses contribute to. Each of us pays a few quid a month into the Mess Fund and in return it keeps us in tea, coffee and toast, and every so often a big fat grand of cash gets put behind a bar and the doctors try to get a few shots in before the nurses steam in and glug back the lot. Although judging by my hangover I appear to have been quite successful last night at kicking those angels into touch.

'At least he didn't throw up, grope any nurses or have sex in the Ladies,' says Louise with a bright white smile, sipping on a Diet Coke at the door. Even dressed in her scrubs Louise is gorgeous. Small and slim, with short dark hair, she is sharp and funny and fantastically clever. This is also her last day in A&E before she goes on to St Thomas's, where she will eventually specialize in maxillo-facial surgery. She is already being groomed for the top, by the slightly sweaty-lipped consultant on the fourth floor, who seems to have quite a line in sexy young Max Foxes (glamorous maxillo-facial girl students) following him around. 'They found two condoms and a Dutch cap on the floor of the toilets this morning,' she declares. Somehow it doesn't sound that grubby coming out of her mouth. 'I know everyone's a bit hot under the collar because it's the end of term, but I would've thought after the dose that went around post the last mess party people might have learnt their lesson.'

'It'll be the physios queuing up for penicillin,' announces Andrea, tapping the side of her nose. 'Mark my words. By the way,' she adds, on her way out of the door, 'the big box of Terry's All Gold in my office is out of bounds. The parents of that young girl with the broken leg who came in over the weekend brought them in last night and I am regifting to Oncology. They don't get many gifts in the cancer ward, so hands off!'

'I am quite happy not to see another chocolate as long as I bloody live,' says Margaret, her hands very much in the air.

'You're safe from me,' says Louise. 'I'm not a Terry's fan.'

You would be amazed by the amount of chocolates that turn up in Andrea's office. As is obvious from the size of her, she is the one who usually takes care of them. It depends where you are in the hospital as to what sort of gifts come your way. The nurses in Maternity get given chocolates but they also get money, as some cultures believe in tipping the midwife, or whoever is around at the time of the birth. Consultants always get champagne. Lots of champagne. I remember Julian telling me that when he worked in IVF for a few months, he got three bottles of Moët in his first two weeks. The senior old boy consultants who have private practices and efficient Rottweiler secretaries always talk about acceptable and unacceptable presents. Whisky is. Gin is not. Wine is. Vodka is not. And champagne is always, obviously, gratefully received. The lovely consultant I was with last year would joke about his wisest cancer patients waiting five years before turning up with a cheque made out to his favourite charitable foundation to say that he had done a good job.

I watch Louise putting her delicious-looking Marks and Spencer lunch in the fridge, and take out my cold sandwich. I am just about to sink my teeth into the dry white crust when a junior doctor comes running into the room. His face is bright red and he is sweating with panic.

'You! And you! Who the hell is on duty here? It's all kicked off in A&E. There's some bloke in reception having a fucking stroke!'

8–9 a.m.

The panic is over by the time I have put my sandwich down, drained my can of Coke and made it into the A&E waiting room. The flapping junior doctor had managed to get most of the department to drop everything and run to his rescue, and the poor bloke having the stroke is totally surrounded by willing and very able pairs of hands and is being wheeled past me straight into an empty bay to be hooked up to the monitors.

Weirdly, strokes are quite a common early-morning presentation. Normally the stroke has occurred at some point in the night and the person wakes up unable to move an arm or a leg. It is, however, quite unusual, I have to admit, for someone actually to have the stroke in the reception. Then again, I have ceased to be shocked and surprised by anything that goes on here.

I poke my head into Andrea's office. She has her broad back to me and is typing away at the computer. She senses me behind her and stretches across a plump left hand to protect the large box of Terry's All Gold on the edge of her desk. I can almost hear her growl. One of the corners is squashed. She clearly hasn't guarded them that well, I think, as someone's already dropped the box on the floor.

'I have eyes in the back of my head,' she declares.

'I am not interested in your chocolates,' I reply.

'Well it's not my body you want,' she says, spinning around in her chair, her hands resting on her round stomach, her short legs crossed at the ankle.

I put on my sweet, vulnerable, butter-wouldn't-melt face. 'I was wondering if you have any paracetamol?'

'That all?' she asks, swiftly opening her top drawer and fishing out a couple of white pills which she then drops into a nearby white paper cup before handing them over. 'You're the third person to ask me this morning.'

'Thanks,' I say, knocking them back in one.

'You need water,' she says.

'Mmm,' I agree, a little too late.

It takes me a couple of eye-watering gagging gulps to get them down.

'How is it so far today?' I ask eventually, wiping my eyes and nodding across towards the A&E waiting room.

'The usual mix,' she shrugs, her back once again to me. 'Someone's already complained that the man with the stroke jumped the queue, so I directed them to the CDU.'

'That is naughty!'

'I know!' She laughs.

The CDU, or clinical decision unit, is where we put people

who are cluttering up A&E. We follow what is known as the Manchester Triage system, which is a way of assessing patients as they arrive in the hospital. The administrations nurse or receptionist notes down the symptoms and gives each patient a colour. Red means you will be seen immediately and is usually something life-threatening. Yellow is serious, but you won't die if you have to wait a bit. Green is minor, and if you are given blue you may as well go home because no one is going to give you the time of day this side of Christmas.

After you have been allocated a colour, the long wait begins. However, due to government guidelines no one is allowed to sit in the A&E waiting room for more than four hours, hence the handy use of the CDU. It is just another place to put patients to sit, a place where there are no time limits to their sitting and no other edicts as to what will happen if they sit there too long. They have officially been processed and are no longer in the A&E system. Some patients, mainly the drunks, are put there for the whole night. It is basically a nice warm place for them to snooze and sober up before we kick them back out into the world in the morning. If you are not drunk and asleep, the CDU is a bad place to be.

'You on with me today?' asks the lovely Louise as she breezes past me.

'Yup.'

'D'you know which consultant?'

'Let's hope it's not Rob,' I reply.

Louise raises her eyebrows and gives me a small nod to show that she understands exactly what I mean.

Rob is charming and nice and great company but he is an

old-school surgeon with a bit of a coke problem. In his early fifties, he was once brilliant and now isn't. He is great to work with, or rather safe to work with, until about lunchtime, then he gets too wired to make much sense and usually has to disappear or be disappeared for the rest of his shift. If he has been up all night, which does happen fairly regularly, he thankfully doesn't come into work at all. He calls in sick, or just doesn't bother to show. In any other walk of life he would have been dismissed long ago, but because he is a consultant and because he was once really rather good, everyone covers for him and he gets paid not to turn up when what he really needs is a kick in the pants and a stint in rehab. But hospitals are littered with people who don't pull their weight. The rarefied world of the consultant means that they answer to few, and just so long as you don't kill anyone and are seen a few days a week walking through the wards with a clipboard and a concerned look on your face, then you're still in business.

I follow Louise into the consultation area. Ours is one of those old Victorian hospitals that really needs knocking down and rebuilding instead of being added to and made over every decade, which is what every successive government has done for the past forty years. We are a big old teaching hospital with such a fine and distinguished reputation that nobody can bear to close or relocate us. So when we need some more space for another department with some more beds, we expand into neighbouring houses or office blocks. What we would all really like is a huge great purpose-built place like the Chelsea and Westminster with an atrium and a carpet and a sexy café meet-and-greet facility, which feels more like a shopping centre than a place for the sick. But, sadly, we are old and buggered and short of space, light, equipment and adequate ventilation. Everything is a bit crap and run down and has seen better days, including A&E. We have ten cordoned-off bays with pale-green curtain divides, and another six to eight private rooms where you can actually close the door. There doesn't seem to be any particular logic to where each patient is put. You would think the more serious the case, the more private the room, but these private rooms are quite hard to get big groups in and out of, so if you are at death's door and awaiting the crash team, the best place to be is a bay. It's quicker to get more hands on the deck and there is significantly more room for people to jump up and down on your chest.

I walk over and check the computer to see who is next in line. Your work rate, or ability to get through the list of in-coming patients, is monitored, so a high and quick turnover is the order of the day. There are some doctors who cheat the system and deliberately choose patients who have been referred to A&E by their GP. They are known as 'medically' or 'clinically expected' and are much easier to deal with than the morass that is the unfiltered general public. Their cases have already been 'worked up' and gone through, which means they slide through the system so much more easily. They do not really qualify as an A&E admission, but once clicked on on the computer system they count as your patient and make you look super-fast and efficient. You can admit them and send them on to the relevant department before your next-door neighbour has even got round to taking his patient's blood pressure.

'This is June,' says Margaret, as I look up from the computer. She takes me by the elbow, hands me a clipboard and ushers me towards an old lady lying on a trolley. 'She is seventy-six years old and fell on a slippery wet pavement this morning on her way to post a letter. She's hurt her hip.'

'Oh, right, thanks.' I look down at the notes and then down at the patient, a rather sweet-looking old lady with a tight grey perm. 'Hello, June,' I say, leaning over and using my special slow and loud old-lady voice. 'I am—'

'I may have fallen over,' she interjects, 'but it hasn't affected my hearing.'

'Oh, I am sorry,' I say, taking a step back and smiling. There's life in the old bird yet, I had better cut the crap. 'Where does it hurt?'

'In my hip.' She winces, shifting on the bed.

I start to feel around the top of her leg as gently as possible. The last thing I want to do is make her feel more uncomfortable than she is. 'How long ago did you do this?'

'About half an hour ago, I think. My neighbour found me in the street. I live on my own, you see.'

'I see.' The joint is already quite swollen, the feeling of a break unmistakable. 'On a scale of one to ten, how bad is the pain?'

'Ten.' She's looking me straight in the eye and I can see she isn't kidding. 'And I have had three children.'

'I am afraid to say that it is a break. I'm not sure how bad just yet but we'll send you up to X-ray and have a look at it.'

She nods.

'Do you have anyone you can call? Someone who can be with you?'

'I think my neighbour is calling my youngest,' she says.

'That's good.' I smile. 'And we'll get you something for the pain.'

I tap the back of her cold, dank, thin hand and her other hand grabs hold of mine.

'Thank you,' she says, both her voice and hands shaking.

I have to say, of all the orthopaedic injuries, a hip fracture is my least favourite, mainly because the outcomes are so poor. There is the terrible statistic that 70 per cent of patients who fracture or break their hip die within two years – something like 1,150 people every month in the UK. This is mainly down to the obvious fact that if you fall and break your hip, your balance and therefore your health cannot be very good. And neither, of course, can your bone density. The other reason hip injuries are so often fatal is that the pain of the fracture means the patient stays in bed, and doesn't move. It hurts too much even to cough, so they don't. The lungs fill with mucus, the mucus breeds bacteria, because bacteria love that sort of shit, and before you know it you have pneumonia. And from there, the only way is down.

I look at June and think about her three children and hope that she is one of the lucky 30 per cent who make it. She looks quite sprightly and with it. Perhaps it was just this shit August drizzle that got her, and not her lack of balance at all.

Margaret disappears off to call the orthopods, or orthopaedic surgeons, to get one of them down for a second look while I fill out an X-ray request form. I am tempted to write down JFDI on the form – just fucking do it – to see if I can get them back any quicker than the usual two hours, but

I think perhaps it's a bit early in the morning to start bullying people. I've a long shift ahead of me and I don't know when I might need to call in a favour.

'Broken hip?' asks Louise as she stands behind me waiting to use the computer.

'Yep,' I say. 'Poor old thing.' I find it quite hard to concentrate when she stands this close to me.

'Christ, we used to get three or four of those a day in Eastbourne.'

'That's OAPs for you.'

'We had nine in one night once.'

'Nine?'

'It was icy and windy. Some old biddy was blown over on the promenade and another was chased by seagulls and fell over.'

'Either that or she had been at the sauce.'

'They're dangerous things, seagulls.' She smiles at me. 'I was attacked by one once, pecked me on the head. I think it was after my fish and chips.'

'How long were you in Eastbourne?'

'Six miserable months in Orthopaedics.'

'Oh yeah.' I nod. 'I remember you saying.'

'I was fresh out of medical school. They were a bunch of tossers in Orthopaedics. I'll never forget one of the surgeons asking who was assisting him in theatre that day, and I put my hand up. He sighed and rolled his eyes and said, "God, I may as well be on my own then."'

'The sexist!' I say.

She looks at me, confused. 'Sexist? No, it was nothing to do with that. It was because I was fresh out of college,' she snaps, picking up her clipboard and bustling past me.

Oh. I stare at her swinging hips as she sashays through A&E. I was just about to tell her about my time in Bognor, at the Bognor Regis War Memorial hospital, when I was also a shiny new junior. All hospitals, despite their specialisms, and the roaming nature of the doctors that populate them, are only ever really a reflection of the community they serve. So, for example, Coventry hospital, because it is at the intersection of the M40, M1, M42, M5 and M6 motorways, was always full of patients who'd had road accidents. Barts and the Royal London, because it's in Whitechapel, is always full of stabbings and shootings. Bognor, as we had Butlins down the road, was constantly having to deal with the fallout from fights between Redcoats and big East End families who'd come in gangs of fifty on holiday. The police had to be called several times to A&E to break up brawls, and on particularly heavy nights we used to have to have security guards keeping the two groups apart.

I finish typing up my notes into June's file, wondering how long she is going to be kept waiting for her X-ray. I am contemplating a quick trip back to the common room to scoff down my bacon sandwich, which I have left on the windowsill by the water-cooler, when I see Louise walking towards me. No sooner has she waltzed off in her feminist huff, I think, than she is straight back. I smile. Her pale blue eyes are looking slightly desperate, like she needs some help.

'Please,' she says, handing me the notes, 'take the bloke in cubicle three.'

'Well . . .' I hesitate.

'I will owe you.'

The idea of Louise owing me something is enough to make me acquiesce to almost anything. 'Yes, of course,' I reply.

'He's got something stuck on his cock,' she says.

'His cock?'

'Yup, some sort of scaffolder's spanner,' she says, walking off in the opposite direction.

'He's a scaffolder?'

'I have no idea,' she says, over her shoulder. 'Thanks, you're a mate.'

I stand behind the pistachio curtain and inhale before drawing it back. 'Morning! And how are we in here?' I look down to see a big bald bloke in his forties, covered in large sailor-blue tattoos, with what looks like a handcuff still attached to one hand. Next to him is standing what I presume to be his wife/girlfriend/partner, dressed in a lemon-yellow T-shirt and pink leggings, with a very concerned expression on her craggy face as she stands over him, mincing her hands. They both smell slightly of old booze.

'Oh doctor,' says the bloke, looking like he is in great pain. 'It's my dick!'

'Right,' I say, pulling back the sheet.

Jesus Christ! I can see what he means. Not only has he got a scaffolder's spanner stuck at the base of his cock but the whole thing has swollen up like a great big red-purple-blue beachball.

'That looks sore,' I say, feeling my legs wanting to cross in sympathy. 'How did you do that?'

'Well . . .' He inhales, then winces. 'You tell 'im, Sheila.'

Sheila shifts from one foot to the next, turns slightly pink, and then goes on to explain that they were having a bit of fun what with this, that and the other when Dave suggested that she put the spanner on the end of his penis and handcuff him and lead him around the house a bit. 'It was all a bit of a laugh, you see,' she says, looking at me through smudged make-up.

'I see,' I say, not really seeing how being led around a room by your cock could ever be a great laugh, but each to their own.

'And then we fell asleep,' says Dave.

'And we woke up to this,' adds Sheila, looking down at Dave's massively engorged penis.

Apparently, the first thing they did was call the fire brigade. They turned up, managed not to laugh, and told him they could take the spanner off but the cock would come too. Obviously deciding that was not the best course of action, they came to A&E.

'OK,' I say. 'I will first of all give you an IV of fluids and a nice strong painkiller and then I think we might have to squeeze your penis a bit and see if we can get that spanner off.'

'OK,' nods Dave, rubbing his handcuffed hand over the top of his bald head, psyching himself up. 'Go ahead, doc.' He pauses. 'I'm not going to lose my dick, am I?'

'Not if I have anything to do with it.' I smile. 'Nurse,' I say, turning to Margaret, who is behind me, doing her best not to laugh, 'IV fluids and—'

'Right away, doctor!' she squeaks before running out of the cubicle.

I am about to march after her, either to accuse her of being unprofessional or have a quick laugh with her, when all hell breaks loose outside in the corridor. There's a lot of shouting and screaming and then a group of four paramedics in green jumpsuits come bursting through the swing doors, wheeling a trolley on which, underneath a blanket, is a writhing, screaming patient.

'Out the way! Out the way! Out the way!' yells a big ginger bloke, pushing and barging people to the left and right. 'Give us some room here!'

I've seen him about before, but never have I seen him looking this goddamn focused.

'Burns!' he barks. 'About forty-five per cent burns!'

Louise and the senior consultant, Mr Williams, who must have literally just arrived for what he thought would be the relaxing early-morning shift, come careering towards me.

'White, male,' continues the ginger paramedic. 'Set fire to himself in Sainsbury's car park at seven thirty this morning—'

'Resus bay,' orders Mr Williams, pointing to the one right next to mine.

'—using petrol. We received the call almost immediately from the security guard who had seen it all on CCTV. We arrived about ten minutes later but not before he'd managed to do himself some serious damage.'

'Fluids?' asks Mr Williams.

'Yup.'

The writhing, screaming man under the blanket is slowly surrounded by more and more nurses and doctors bringing fluids and painkillers and bandages. He must be very miserable indeed, I think, walking over to the other side of the department in search of a baby blood pressure cuff. He has done himself some serious damage; 45 per cent is life-threatening. Actually, any burn can be life-threatening, it just depends on how young and well you are to start off with. A month ago we had a ninety-eight-year-old woman in with a small burn, 11 to 12 per cent. She'd got it in the bath. The hot tap was running and she was too old and frail to turn it off, and she got stuck in there. Eventually she was found by a carer and was brought in. The terrible thing was, even as I examined her, I knew she wasn't going to survive. She was too old for us to operate on, because the anaesthetic would kill her, and if we didn't operate on her she would die. And she did. It took a couple of weeks. She slipped away. Slowly but surely she got weaker and weaker. It was very depressing to watch. I did go and see her, and every day I talked to her a bit more, and every day she talked to me a little less.

We get quite a few of those types of domestic burns in here. Small children who have spilt hot cups of tea or coffee over themselves. We had three members of one family come in last week because the grandfather had decided to put some liquid accelerant on a barbecue that was already alight. The wind blew and the flames went all over his daughter and two grand-children. They were 30 per cent burns.

There are three types of burn: accident, assault and self-immolation. Bizarrely, people setting fire to themselves due to depression is the most common cause of major burns. Although we have had a spate recently of very burnt drug addicts who were all stealing copper piping. As the price of copper increases, so does its scrap value; the only problem is that when these guys steal it they forget that there is usually gas running through it and it blows up in their faces. We have had three in the last two months.

By the time I get back to my cubicle, Margaret's great big morphine shot has clearly worked its magic because Sheila has left the area and Dave is fast asleep, with his swollen cock hanging out for all to see. I take a deep breath, snap on a surgical glove and take a firm hold of his penis. I massage and squeeze, trying to encourage the blood back down, through the spanner. Dave starts to moan. I can only hope it's through pain and not pleasure.

Next door, I can hear the resus team battling to help the screaming burns victim. There are monitors bleeping, and the sound of dressing packets being torn open. I look down and stop tugging. Dave's penis seems a little bit smaller, although his snores are getting louder. I get out the baby blood pressure cuff, wrap it around the blue/red member and start to pump it up. Over the little hissing noises, I hear Dave break wind.

Why is it that I always get the glory jobs?

9–10 a.m.

I have to say I'm not sure who is more relieved when the spanner finally comes off, Dave or me. Dave is obviously chuffed that he hasn't actually lost his cock after one night of fooling around with his missus, and I am only too delighted not to have to tug and massage another man's penis any longer than is actually necessary. Dave hasn't got off scot-free, though, as he'll be out of action for a while, waiting for the swelling to go down completely and the sensation to return. However, one thing is certain: he will now be slightly more circumspect when it comes to bringing his work tools home with him.

'Sorry about that,' says Louise as she comes out of the resus cubicle, wiping away a strand of sweaty dark hair with the back of a gloved hand. 'It's just I had to squeeze a penis for over an hour at the weekend after the tip had become so engorged the foreskin couldn't get over the end of it. It was tight around the end of the knob like some rubber band.'

'Right,' I say, trying to put the painful and at the same time extremely pleasurable image out of my mind.

'Anyway, the man was remarkably ungrateful,' she says.

'The fool.' I laugh.

'He was more than that,' she responds, her brown eyes narrowing. 'I practically got repetitive strain injury.' She holds up her hand and simulates the move.

All I can think of is her lucky, lucky boyfriend.

'How's it going in there?' I ask, swiftly changing the subject, looking over her shoulder at the now quiet burns man who is almost completely swaddled in bandages.

'Ba-a-ad,' she whispers. 'Fifty-fifty I'd say. Mr Williams has put a call in to Plastics to see if they can do anything to make him more comfortable.'

'I presume he meant to do it?'

'He's not saying. I'm not sure he can speak at the moment, he's in shock.'

She walks off. I wander over to the doors to the waiting room. I can see through the glass panels that the place is beginning to fill up with the usual sprains and tumbles as the real world gets out of bed, has its breakfast, buys its newspapers and heads off to work. Judging by the number of falls down stairs, slips in the shower and trips over the dog we get at this time in the morning, getting up is a hazardous process indeed.

Come nine a.m., along with those who find getting to work a little difficult, we also start to get the lonely. There is normally a collection of old ladies who like to use the cosy confines of the A&E waiting room as a bit of a drop-in centre. Some of them wake up, realize they are not going to see anyone all day, so get themselves all dressed up and off to A&E for a chat, a cup of tea and a biscuit, which is what the nurses give them for making the effort to come in. Others call an ambulance. Not something we encourage, obviously, as an ambulance costs around £800 a pop, but somehow it's hard to get cross with them. Around lunchtime there is normally quite a gathering. They tend to favour the far corner of the waiting room, near the table covered in crumpled magazines, where they pile up the free newspapers. It's closest to the telly. And they all quite like a bit of Jeremy Kyle with their Rich Tea. I can see a couple of them already ensconced in the corner, thick coats and glasses on. They look settled in for the day.

I walk up to the desk in the corner of the department, next to the door of Andrea's office. I wait for a few minutes for Ewan, a fellow senior house officer, to finish up. Mr Williams is sitting half-buttocked on the desk, on the phone.

'Can you bloody believe it,' he says to either or both of us, as he covers the receiver with his hand. 'I have been on hold for seven minutes now while they try and track down a plastic bloody surgeon to come look at our burns bloke. I mean, what else are they supposed to be doing up there? Dolly Parton's tits?'

'I think those might have been done already,' I suggest.

'What?' he says, looking at me as if for the first time.

'Dolly Parton's tits?'

'Yes, yes,' he says, rustling some papers in front of him. 'Also I couldn't park this morning. There are just not enough spaces for the consultants.'

And their big fat cars, I think. I don't know what it is about consultants and their cars, but as soon as they get their consultancy they feel the need to embrace their inner pimp and buy themselves a ridiculous set of shut-up-and-look-at-my-cock wheels. The hospital car park is full of them. Half of those motors wouldn't look out of place at Old Trafford – there are Porsches, Mercs, BMWs and a very tasty collection of Maseratis. Most of the consultants easily clear over £150,000 a year working for the NHS alone, not including private practice, so it isn't surprising they can afford to shell out on fancy cars. But they all seem to think they have to. And they also park so badly. When I worked in Bognor there was a swinging-dick surgeon who used to park his red Porsche on the yellow zigzags outside A&E. There is a culture of not wanting consultant surgeons to come into the hospital in a bad mood, so they are allowed to park how and where they like.

The parking pisses everyone off here, especially the relatives who want to come and visit. Not only do they have to pay, earning the NHS £110 million a year in fees, but there is never anywhere to put your vehicle. The main problem is that the visiting hours are the same for every ward on the hospital, so everyone arrives and leaves at the same time. If only visiting times were staggered, that would in turn stagger the pressure on the visitors' car park. It seems so simple. But nothing is ever simple here. In fact, mention parking at the beginning of an hour-long meeting in this building and it would be the only thing discussed.

'So I've popped the Beemer on some double yellows round the back,' announces Mr Williams.

'Right,' says Ewan. 'I'm sure it'll be fine there.'

'Mmm.' He pauses. 'So, have you guys thought about fundraising ideas for the Da Vinci Robot?'

'Do we really need one?' says Ewan.

'Of course we do!' says Mr Williams, looking shocked that Ewan doesn't think that over £1.2 million of surgical equipment is a must-have in these cash-strapped times. Pioneered in London and developed and manufactured in California, the Da Vinci Robot is a means of carrying out extreme tremor-free microsurgery, and Mr Williams is clearly of the view that any hospital worth its subsidy should have one. 'Guildford's got one, for Chrissake.'

'I think Alison's going off there tomorrow,' says Ewan.

'What, Alison with the double D-cup?' queries Mr Williams.

A senior consultant and a real A&E pro, Chris Williams is lean and fit, with brown hair that is turning steely-grey at the temples. He is great in a crisis, capable of cracking a chest on a trolley and delivering a baby in a lift. He is knocking fifty and very much old-school. He always says that he trained when doctors were real men and they had to do a thousand-hour week, drink fifteen pints of vodka and still sleep with all the nurses. He has a good line in banter and is a great favourite with the old ladies, but he is also a talented surgeon, and no one can work out why he isn't making a fortune in the private sector and is still flogging his guts out in A&E. Perhaps he enjoys the rush? Just as other consultants love being called off the golf course, or out of their child's first birthday party, for an urgent life-saving operation – maybe it's the need to be needed that rocks his boat? Or maybe he's just really old-fashioned and likes helping people. All I know is that he is an A&E specialist and he is one of the best, even if he is a little bit lascivious around the edges.

'Fuck it,' says Chris, suddenly getting off the desk, 'I'm too busy for this. Take it.' He hands the receiver to Ewan. 'And tell them when they have finished making a seventy-five-year-old banker's wife look twelve that we'd like someone down here to check out the grade three burns on my patient to see if we can do anything for him tonight or if we can book him in for an op tomorrow. OK?'

'OK.' Ewan nods, picking up the phone. 'Do you want any surgeon in particular?'

'Nope,' says Chris, disappearing off down a corridor. 'Just get through to bloody someone.'

Ewan busies himself holding the phone and picking his ear, while I briefly type in a few notes about Dave's tremendously swollen cock. Then, just as I am finishing up, I look over the computer at the door to Andrea's office, which is slightly ajar. Through the crack, I recognize the blonde bobbing head of Margaret, who seems to be on her knees with her face embedded in a pair of trousers. I give Ewan a whack in the gut to get his attention.

'Jesus,' he says as he looks over, the scene slowly dawning on him. 'It's a bit early for that.'

'Last day of term, I suppose,' I say with a grin as I try to work out who is being relieved so pleasurably in what is effectively matron's office.

Ewan and I are still watching when the door swings open a little more to reveal Steve looking straight back at us, zipping up his fly. A good-looking SHO from Manchester who is moving back up north to specialize in paediatrics, he is always lucky with the ladies.

'Ah, great! There you are, Margaret,' booms Chris's voice from behind me.

Margaret leaps up and turns around rather red-faced, running her hands through her hair. The blonde strands that normally fall forward suddenly appear slicked back. She looks extremely sheepish. Fortunately, Chris is too distracted to notice.

'Your hair is looking good,' he says.

I look at Steve, who turns puce, and Ewan, who bites the side of his cheek. I can't begin to catch Margaret's eye.

'Thanks,' she somehow manages to say.

'Now,' Chris continues, 'this is Mr Berry and he is our new A&E manager. He used to work with Asda so he is very qualified to look after us lot.' He tugs at a clump of his greying hair and looks towards the heavens for some sort of intervention or explanation. 'Anyway, Mr Berry, this is Margaret, one of our best nurses. She'll show you around the place.'

'Hello, Mr Berry,' says Margaret, her hair glistening in the neon strip light.

'Please, call me Jon,' he says, rocking back and forth on the thick soles of his Hush Puppies.

'OK then, Jon,' says Margaret, clawing back some dignity. 'Let's start with the A&E waiting room.'

Margaret escorts the suited Jon Berry down the corridor.

'He looks about fourteen,' says Chris, sounding deeply depressed. 'Well, he can't be any worse than that last woman.'

The 'last woman' was a total cow with a penchant for megalomania. She would march up and down the corridor in her power suit, with her power shoes, sporting her power specs, issue orders while waving a clipboard and demand to know why this patient was sitting on a trolley in the corridor, or why that patient was still waiting after four and a half hours. What we wanted to do was shout in her power ear that we were 'too fucking short-staffed' or 'too fucking busy' and 'if we could fucking do something about it we fucking would'. Obviously we would have ended up the subject of some sort of disciplinary action, in some sort of committee room. So we lied. Not great big porkie pies. Just little ones. We didn't exactly hide patients from her but just fibbed about how long they had been waiting, and what they were waiting for. 'Waiting for a chest X-ray' was one of my favourites. That usually got rid of her for an hour, before she'd trot back on her high horse looking to find fault.

We took a bit of badgering initially. We were all keen to improve the department and up our stats. But then we'd get memos like the one that complained we were spending too much money on 'staffing, consumables and drugs'. We were a hospital that was spending too much on doctors, nurses and things that make people better! Unbelievable. She then asked Andrea to write a report to the director of operations to explain why our deaths per week were up and our performance had dropped since October. She was given one hour to write it, which seemed a little unprofessional, and indeed unfair.

But management just loves to tick a box or fill in a form. The four-hour A&E waiting time edict just means that there are a lot of patients admitted into the hospital who shouldn't be there. Better to shove them on a ward somewhere to get them out of the way and then if we are really smart we can process them and get them out again within twenty-three hours, so another target is hit: people who spend less than a day in hospital. Who cares if they spend another six hours in the 'discharge lounge', just so long as we can use their still-warm bed? Or indeed another five hours sitting in the hospital pharmacy waiting for their take-home meds? We've hit all our targets. The government will be ever so pleased and we can have some more money. And woe betide any hospital that gets a surgeon or a physician who is a maverick genius. What the system wants is doctors or surgeons who go nicely down their lists and clear their decks and keep as few people waiting as possible. The problem with the genius doctors is that they attract more 'clients', or patients; people start choosing to come to your hospital, and then you are in all sorts of trouble. Your waiting lists grow longer and your stats go down. No, no, no, talent, flair and brilliance are absolutely not to be encouraged.

'I hope he's got a better degree than her, though,' adds Chris as he turns to go back and check on his burns patient. 'She had a two-two in business administration from Kettering

University. And you,' he says to Steve, 'had better put your scrubs on. You're due on at ten a.m.'

I follow Steve along the corridor, as I am now desperate for my bacon sandwich. The fact that it will be not only cold but congealed now is only adding to its allure, I am that goddamn hungry.

'D'you think I got away with that?' asks Steve.

'What, morally, emotionally? Or, did Chris clock what was going on?'

'Mr Williams, of course.'

'Don't think he saw anything.'

'Really?'

'Not that I noticed,' I say.

'Excellent,' sniffs Steve. 'Maggie's been promising me one for the last six months and, you know, last day and all that . . .'

'Carpe diem, mate, carpe diem,' I say, heading off to the common room and my sandwich.

'My thoughts exactly,' he says, going into the changing room.

The common room is already filling up with the detritus of the day. There are crisp packets on the floor, sweet papers on the chairs, and the air has that slightly sweet, cloying smell of McDonald's chips. I look around on the windowsill for my bacon sandwich but it seems to have disappeared. Shit! I check the next-door windowsill and the floor around it just in case someone's knocked it off. Shit! It's been pinched. Either that or thrown away. But no one clears up this place, least of all the cleaners. About once a month the fridge gets emptied of all the rotting half-eaten packed lunches, but that's only for health and safety reasons. No one would tidy up a sandwich.

I am livid. I can feel a wave of indignity and injustice rising in me. My stomach grumbles with self-pity. Two can play at the game, I think, striding towards the fridge. I check in the door. Quite frankly, anything that is in the fridge door is fair game. Everyone knows that. You would have to be an idiot, or new, to put anything unopened in the door. Oh my God, joy of joys! Half a KitKat! I grab the two fingers with both hands, shove them straight in, and make a very sharp exit.

With my cheeks fuller than a hamster preparing for a famine, I walk back out into the corridor and bump slap-bang into Andy, an anaesthetist who has a bit of a charm-bypass problem.

'All right?' he asks. 'I hear you made a bit of a dick of yourself last night.'

Andy is typical of a myriad of anaesthetists who appear to follow the ABCD rule as they attend a crash call. They Arrive, Bitch, Criticize, then Depart. The theory is that because all they ever really have to worry about is their tray of syringes and what order to use them in – big syringe, little syringe, or little syringe, big syringe? – they have plenty of time to stick their long noses into other people's business. And if they aren't bitching, they are sitting on their gas tanks doing the *Times* crossword, or sudoku, depending on their age. There are a few of them who are quite cool; after all, they are experts on using all sorts of drugs from opiates to mind-bending hallucinogens, and they get paid £100,000 a year for their trouble. But it is an odd job – 90 per cent boredom, 10 per cent life-threatening fear – and it does seem to attract quite an odd bunch of people.

Most of them choose it as their specialism because you have a regular lifestyle, others because they have an OCD about achieving the perfect take-off and landing – i.e. the perfect way to put someone to sleep and wake them up again. But there are others, like Andy, who do it because they are dull twunts with no bedside manner at all.

'Really?' I say, slightly wanting to kick him in the blue-scrubbed nuts. 'What did you hear?'

'That you were dancing in a wig,' he sniggers.

'Right.'

'And that you were really drunk,' he adds, for good measure.

'At least I wasn't sitting on my own with a Diet Coke.'

'I had to work today,' he says defensively.

'And I am here for my health.' I start to walk away.

'Ha ha,' he says. 'But some of us take our jobs seriously.'

'Go and put someone to sleep, Andy. Actually, why don't you talk to them and save yourself some drugs?'

'Did you hear Louise was caught in a linen cupboard with Mr Williams?' he declares.

I stop in my tracks.

'There!' he says. 'That woke you up!'

'Don't believe you.'

'Ask her yourself, seeing as you two are such good mates!' And with that he walks off in the direction of the operating theatre.

Louise? And Mr Williams? Chris? But he's married. Second wife, I grant you. And he has four children. Surgeons always have lots of children. I'm not sure if it's because they live such a visceral existence, or they think their genes need to be replicated as much as possible. I met a surgeon once who proudly announced that his genes were so goddamn marvellous that he needed to have three children with three different wives. (God administered a certain cruel justice in the end: his third wife had twins and he was taken out by a massive stroke soon after they were born.) Typical surgeon behaviour – all about targets.

'Oh there you are,' says Louise, running up to me in the corridor.

'Sorry,' I say, rather embarrassed at being busted thinking about her sex life. 'Um, how can I help you?'

'Please don't be cross,' she says, smiling sweetly and ruffling her short dark hair. 'But I told Mr Williams you would do it.'

'Do what?'

'You were so good at the last one.'

'Which last one?'

'There's a poor bloke in there with priapism.'

My heart sinks.

'He is best man at a wedding at two p.m. and he's desperate. He has tried water, ice, Ann Widdecombe . . .' She smiles again.

'Go on then,' I say. 'You may as well just call me Dr Cock.'

'Actually, *Mr* Cock, seeing as you're a surgeon,' she says, linking her arm in mine and walking up the corridor with me. 'And can I just warn you, it is enormous!'

10–11 a.m.

Louise is not joking. It is not the largest I have seen by a long way, but the bloke is certainly gifted. And, of course, mortified. Priapism is caused by many things – neurological dysfunction, spinal cord lesions, even reactions to drugs or a spider bite – but the most common reasons are sickle cell anaemia and Viagra.

We have had a few Viagra overdoses in recently. Most were treatable. Even when one of our paediatric surgeons came in after a heavy weekend with his wife, we mostly managed to treat the penis by sticking a needle in it and aspirating away the blood. But we had one bloke in a few months ago which was a complete disaster. His girlfriend had gone away for a week and he had shipped in a whole load of Viagra and an extra-curricular girl. I'm not sure if she was a prostitute or another girlfriend, all I know is that she didn't stick around to witness the fallout. Anyway, his erection didn't go down after the weekend. I'm not sure if it was because he was embarrassed per se or whether it was guilt about being unfaithful that stopped him coming in. But he didn't come in until the Wednesday, which was a huge mistake. By the time he got to us, his penis had turned black. It was black and rock hard. The blood that was stuck in the end of it had congealed and hardened. His cock was effectively dead. We tried to massage the thing, cannulate it, fill it full of fluid, revive it in any way, but that was it. It was solid and therefore dead. So the girl-friend came back after a week of being away to find out that not only had her boyfriend been unfaithful, he had lost his cock in the process.

Fortunately, this bloke has only had an erection since about seven this morning, he doesn't have sickle cell anaemia, and neither has he been using Viagra. However, that does not make him any less desperate. Going through his notes and talking to him, it transpires that he has suffered from the condition before, and it tends to get worse when he is nervous. Obviously being best man this afternoon has brought the condition on. I offer him a drug to help bring the problem under control but it will be too slow-acting for him to make the wedding. He even contemplates going to the service and then coming back to hospital before the reception, but his trousers and boxer shorts can't contain his 'excitement' and it is extremely obvious what is going on. So he looks at me and I look at him and then he says, 'Go on, doc, do your worst.' I explain to him that a nurse and I will each put a large needle into the shaft and attempt to take out as much blood as we can, to see if we can make the thing go down. I have to say his face falls a little when he sees Andrea arrive, from behind the curtains, bearing a syringe. Despite the local anaesthetic he screams the place down – which is not that helpful when you have a room full of patients waiting. Then again, you can hardly blame him. It has to be one of our more painful procedures.

It does the trick, though. Ten minutes later he is all smiles and hugs as he gets back into his clothes and sprints off to pick up his morning suit.

Back at the computer, I am standing next to Chris Williams waiting for Jon Berry to finish whatever important bit of 'management' he is doing.

'How long was Mr Johnson waiting?' Jon Berry asks over the top of his short sweaty nose.

'Who?' I ask.

'Your last patient?'

'The one with the huge erection?' I say, to wind him up a little. I can see Chris smiling behind him.

'That's the one,' Jon Berry responds, completely unfazed.

'Forty-two minutes.'

'Excellent,' he says, typing away.

Chris gives me a quizzical look and I shrug back. It was a figure I plucked from nowhere. He wasn't my patient, he was Louise's; she clicked on him on the computer. But the number sounded plausible and, most importantly, very efficient.

'Talking of cocks,' injects Chris – which we weren't – 'did you hear what happened last week at the Orthopaedic Surgeons Golf Dinner?'

'No?' I say. 'And anyway, what were you doing there?'

'My mate Jeff is getting divorced and I play off twelve, so I was his plus one.'

'Is that good?' I ask.

'Very. Don't you play golf?' Chris sounds somewhat incredulous.

'No.'

'How are you going to get on!' It was more of a statement than a question.

I look a little uncomfortable. Clearly, being a good surgeon is not enough.

'Anyway,' continues Chris, 'there's this one orthopod who had a sex change, the whole thing, the full penis-off, man-in-a-boat exchange—'

'Man in a boat?' asks Jon Berry.

'A clitoris, man, a clitoris!' says Chris, irritated at the interruption. 'He was married, you know, two children. Anyway, that's not a problem. If a man wants to be a woman, then good luck to him. No. What really pissed us all off was that he teed off with the ladies. I mean, the balls of it! Or, indeed, lack of. But, really! He won, obviously. Quite ruined everyone's afternoon.'

'I can imagine,' I say, trying my hardest to empathize.

Jon Berry just sits there, typing away, his ears throbbing red with embarrassment.

'Is the new doctor here yet?' Chris interjects suddenly by way of covering the silence.

I look at him blankly.

'Mr Lee. The one from China, he is supposed to be arriving today? He should be here by now.'

We both look back past the computer and into A&E. The place is buzzing. Most of the cubicles are occupied, there are nurses bustling briskly to and fro, Steve is helping an elderly woman who appears to have a large bruise on her head into a chair, Louise has a fistful of bloods and is making her way over to the chute, Ewan looks to have his hands full with some screaming child and his equally uncooperative mother, Margaret's hair is a little less shiny as she wheels an IV stand across the corridor, and Andrea is standing by her office door, chewing a toffee, guarding her chocolates.

'I can't see him,' I say.

'Yes, well,' says Chris. 'Tell me if you do. And come and get me when Buggerlugs here is off the computer.'

'You can't call me that,' says Jon Berry, indignantly.

'So sack me!' says Chris, walking away.

'One surgeon was fired recently for putting extra croutons on his salad and not paying for them,' replies Jon Berry, by way of a weak threat.

'I never eat in the canteen,' retorts Chris, before disappearing behind a pistachio curtain.

I am just about to check with Andrea that June, with the broken hip, has been taken off to X-ray – as her cubicle now appears to be empty – and if they have room for her upstairs, when I spot Mr Lee wandering into the department. Short, definitely under five foot, he has thick specs and an even thicker girth. He is smiling broadly – I'm not sure whether out of friendliness or bewilderment.

'Mr Lee!' I say, walking towards him with my hand outstretched. 'Welcome to A&E!'

He smiles at me and hesitantly takes my hand. I shake it. He shakes back and bows his head slightly, muttering under his breath.

'You stay there and I'll go and find Mr Williams for you.'

He smiles at me again and I smile back and walk off to find out which pistachio curtain Mr Williams is hiding behind. Mr Lee follows me. I interrupt Ewan looking down the mouth of his moaning child. In the next cubicle I find Chris shining a torch into the eyes of a man who has been splashed in the face with some unpleasant chemical at work.

'I am sorry to interrupt,' I begin, 'but Mr Lee is here.'

'Excellent, excellent,' says Chris, peeling back the poor bloke's eyelids just that bit further. 'You seem to be OK. I'll get one of the nurses to give them a rinse, then we'll get you a nice cream to dull the pain for a few days, and you should be fine.' Chris squeezes the bloke's shoulder and he smiles appreciatively. 'Ah! Now, Mr Lee!' he exclaims, turning around to shake the doctor's hand. 'How are you? How was your journey? When did you arrive?'

Chris fires off questions as he ushers the diminutive Mr Lee down the corridor away from the patients and towards Andrea's office and the computer desk. Mr Lee nods away and smiles at everything. By the time Chris reaches the desk it begins to dawn on both him and me that Mr Lee has not answered a single question or even uttered a word. Chris pauses and runs his hands through his grey temple hair.

'Um, Mr Lee, I hope you don't mind me asking . . .'

Mr Lee nods.

'Can you actually speak any English?'

We all look down at the tiny bloke, who looks back up at us, and smiles again. 'Chinese,' he says, finally. 'Chinese.'

'English?' asks Chris.

'Oh.' He nods. 'Google translate.'

'Google translate?' asks Chris.

'Google translate,' he confirms.

'But I have been emailing the man for months,' says Chris. 'Asking him questions, saying that we were looking forward to having him in the department, sharing our knowledge and all that jazz, and he has replied in perfect English every time.'

'English?' Mr Lee nods again. 'Google translate.'

'Google bloody translate!' declares Chris.

'You just type in what you want to say and it translates it,' explains Jon Berry from the computer.

'I know what it does!' says Chris. 'What it means is we have paid for the flight, board and lodging of someone who can't communicate with a single patient!'

Not that being able to speak English appears to be a priority in the NHS any more when it comes to hiring doctors. As members of the European Community we opened our doors to foreign doctors who can practise here without having to sit exams or pass language fluency tests. Only those who live outside the EU have to sit the PLAB (Professional and Linguistic Assessment Board) tests, which means that it is much harder for the NHS to recruit in its old Commonwealth stamping grounds of India, Australia and South Africa, where ironically the inhabitants already speak English, and have been trained in the UK system, or something similar. The result is that the UK is no longer the ultimate destination for doctors all over the world.

After the Red Army, the Indian Railways and, I think now, Wal-Mart, the NHS is the largest employer in the world and it used to be a Mecca for all aspiring doctors, as unlike many other health services in the world it does not promote nationals over foreign doctors. Once you are accepted into the NHS community, you can rise through its ranks, specialize and get a consultancy, no matter where you came from. It is a remarkably egalitarian place to work; your rights and duties are the same as any other doctor within the system. No one will say 'You're from Nigeria, you can't become an ear, nose and throat specialist.' Whereas in other countries, even in the EU, they will train and promote their own doctors above others, and even make sure that some of the more lucrative specialisms, such as ENT or facial plastics, are not open to foreign doctors. I had a friend who was born in Damascus who found it impossible to be an ophthalmic surgeon in the US. The only options open to him were paediatrics, general medicine, anaesthesia and pathology – none of which is a big earner, which is why he was allowed to do them.

You'd be amazed what actually are the big cash jobs within the health service. It is not necessarily the big jobs that earn the big money. What you need in order to earn money in medicine is a high turnover. Quick ops that are low-risk and don't take much time. Things like cataracts, which used to be difficult but are now quick and easy and, at a grand a pop, a very good line of work to get into. It's the old widget factory idea. There's an operation called a stapedectomy, which involves taking a small bone out of the ear and replacing it with a tiny piston, which is quite handy. It takes three minutes and earns the surgeon

£500 a go. A colonoscopy is also quite useful. It's an anal and lower gut examination that takes about twenty minutes; the hospital gets a grand for each one, and the consultant pockets about £300. There are hernia clinics which charge over a couple of grand per hernia. The surgeon will probably get about £300 to £400 per operation. And he will, obviously, be doing a few of those a day.

There are also the backhanders that doctors get for recommending certain consultants. Say I have a patient who needs a cancerous lump removed from her thyroid. There are numerous ENT specialists I can choose from, but if I have a friend who promises to give me 10 per cent of the fee then why not recommend him? Specialist consultants can't lobby for patients, they are totally dependent on referrals, which puts them at the unscrupulous mercy of others further down the food chain. And the more specialized and rarefied they are, the more isolated they are from their 'clients', therefore the more dependent they are on referrals from their generous colleagues. It is an odd situation.

Also, you have to remember that the world of medicine is not static; what has feathered a surgeon's nest nicely for a decade can suddenly change. Bypass grafts used to be the big earner for cardiac surgeons. They would work all day in the NHS, then come six p.m. they'd pop out and do two or three private bypasses at £5,000 each. No wonder, then, that plenty of the big boys were on a million-plus a year. Sadly, statins have ruined that little business. Peptic ulcers also used to be lucrative. It was easy to take things out of stomachs. It didn't take long and wasn't tricky, and plenty of people had bleeding ulcers, perforated ulcers, peptic ulcers. Now, of course, they are all treated by pills.

And the amount of money charged is all so random. No one is really terribly sure why an eye op is £2,500 and a knee op is £1,500. It all boils down to what the insurance companies are prepared to pay. The same goes for the price of a hospital room. The cost of a night in a private hospital or of a private room in a NHS hospital is more or less plucked out of the ether. The overheads, rent and servicing in a NHS hospital are already taken care of – so the £1,000 bill is entirely fictitious. It sounds about the going rate, so it becomes the going rate. No one anywhere can tell you the reason why.

Not that doctors become doctors to make money. I became a doctor because my father was one and his father was one before him. It's a family business, as it were, and to say that I was channelled in that direction would be an understatement. I had a skeleton on my bedroom wall as a child and could name all the bones by the time I was seven years old. My dad is a GP and he has a small but grateful practice just outside Reigate. Sadly, he is not one of the four thousand or so GPs who earn 'more than the Prime Minister' – like that is the litmus test of importance or indeed value for money. But he does quite nicely, thank you. Having said that, when you hear of some GPs earning over £400,000 a year, you do have to question the system that cuts their working hours by seven hours a week and gives them bonuses for treating certain patients, and results in one savvy spark, Dr Shiverdorayi Raghavan, trousering over a million quid from the NHS in two years from his two Birmingham surgeries.

But in general, doctors don't make big money on the NHS. They make a tidy £100,000 and have quite a nice pension as well, but the real money is elsewhere. A surgeon mate of my dad's who has a large private ENT practice says that he spends four-fifths of his time working for the NHS for one-fifth of his income. His set-up is the Shangri-La for doctors – working for the NHS and having a healthy private practice at the same time. Doctors who ditch the NHS completely in order whole-heartedly to chase the dollar are always viewed poorly by their own profession. Firstly, there is an old-fashioned residual idea that you were trained by the NHS, therefore you owe the system and need to pay it back. And secondly, it is only working within the NHS that you get to do the big operations and learn about the new techniques and hear about the new medical advances. If you are out of the system you tend to fall behind. Mainly because you can't afford to do the big operations as your facilities aren't state-of-the-art and your support staff aren't trained highly enough and you can't afford the insurance. You can only do the big stuff at the big teaching hospitals, as they are the only places that have properly staffed intensive care units to look after the patients.

These days, of course, with so many of us doctors sloshing about, private practices are as difficult to come by as consultancy posts. And they are also regional. Only 10 to 11 per cent of the population have private medical insurance, which obviously means that the other 90 per cent do not. So if you want to work in private practice you need to be in the right catchment areas. Jobs and practices in London and the south-east are therefore contested more fiercely than those without a private practice in the north. There was a story going about last year that a plastic surgery patient wreaked revenge on his surgeon for a botched skin graft job by shooting him. Other plastics guys immediately got on the phone, not to send flowers or their condolences, but to find out where the bloke worked. A vacancy is a vacancy after all.

There are plenty of drawbacks to private practice. It is not all plain sailing towards the £900,000-a-year pay cheque. There's the £50,000-a-year-plus insurance to pay, as well as the dreary droning on from the clients to put up with. I have a friend who is a neurologist who has several email accounts so that he is not inundated by the 'worried well'. He gives out certain accounts to certain people who he knows might need a little bit more of his time than others. The attention seekers might find him abroad more often than is strictly the truth, or just that little bit more elusive than other less demanding patients. Private patients call whenever they like, you see. Most think nothing of calling at three a.m. to discuss a headache. My friend says the more they pay, the more they like to talk.

And, interestingly, as more women are becoming doctors, lifestyle is starting to play a part in the popularity of practices. Whereas before the glamour jobs such as cardiac surgery and plastics were the ones that were oversubscribed, now suddenly the jobs with more sociable hours are topping the lists. Dermatology is currently a favourite. There are very few emergency dermatological call-outs, and the rest of the time you are dealing with patients who make appointments with excellent private practice potential.

Right now I have a feeling that Chris Williams is rather wishing that he had a private practice to retire to this morning, rather than deal with the diminutive Mr Lee and his inability to understand a bloody word anyone is saying to him. Chris is on the phone to Administration, admonishing them for hiring someone he himself had personally vouched for. While the rest of us try to avoid the prying eyes of Jon Berry and his increasingly persistent questions and dull fascination for four-hour waiting times.

I have just managed to sidestep his advances and am on my way to grab a swig of water from the cooler in the corner when the double doors crash open and an ambulance crew come steaming in. Chris drops the phone and comes running, grabbing my arm as he passes.

'You!' he says.

I follow him into the resus cubicle. The patient, a woman, doesn't appear to be moving. Her thick blonde hair curls off the trolley in wet clumps; beneath her oxygen mask her mouth is hanging open. When I worked in Geriatrics for six long months, we used to joke about patients lying in bed with their mouths open. There was the 'O-sign': the mouth was open and round, which meant that they were alive, just. Then the 'Q-sign', when the mouth was open and the tongue was hanging to one side. They were dead. And then the 'T-sign', which was the number of undrunk cups of tea sitting beside the bed, which was indicative of how long they had been dead. This woman has an O-sign, which is not good, but obviously better than a Q.

There are two ambulance crew with her, who are filling

Chris, Margaret and me in as we check her over, give her fluids
and wire her up to the machines.

'What's her name?' I ask.

'Rebecca, Rebecca Benson,' replies the tallest bloke, with a
two-day beard.

'Hello, Rebecca? Can you hear me? Rebecca? Can you hear
me? You're in hospital, Rebecca. If you can hear me, Rebecca,
say something.'

She is pretty, in her early thirties I would say.

'Take my hand, Rebecca. Give it a squeeze if you can hear
me.'

Her hands are slim and her fingernails are painted pale pink.
She's wearing a wedding ring and a diamond engagement
ring.

I pull back her dark curling lashes. Her pupils are blown.
They are not responsive to my torch at all. 'Can you hear me,
Rebecca? Squeeze my hand.' Nothing. She does nothing. She
just lies there. She is breathing on her own, but only just. The
chances of asphyxia are high. 'Tube her?' I ask.

Chris nods.

According to the ambulance guys she fell out of the back of
a boat as she was going waterskiing this morning and hit her
head as she entered the water. Her heart stopped. They've
administered CPR but they are not sure how long a downtime
she has had. Chris pulls back the blanket to look at her chest.
She is wearing the remains of a wetsuit which has been pulled
back to reveal a yellow bikini top. Her bosom is a mass of red
and purple bruising. They tried their best, but sometimes these
guys literally punch your chest in order to get your heart

beating. But at least her heart is now working; it's the down-time that's the problem.

'How long was she down for do you think?' asks Chris, checking her over for any signs of life.

'The on-site medic at the reservoir had already started CPR when we got there,' says the taller member of the ambulance crew. 'He said about three to four minutes.'

'You sure?' says Chris, running a pen the length of the soles of her feet; her pink painted toes don't curl. He sticks the point of the pen into her leg. Still nothing. 'It feels longer to me; she's not very responsive. What do you think?' he asks me.

I look at her slim, active-looking yet lifeless body and I feel my heart sink a little. 'I think we'll only really know after the CT scan. It's hard to tell otherwise.'

'But in your gut?'

'Over five.'

'Let's hope she believes in God,' says Chris, scratching his grey hair. 'Because she is sure as hell going to need him now.'

11 a.m.–12 p.m.

Margaret and I accompany Rebecca Benson and two porters up to the intensive care unit. They are two agency nurses short this morning and it's quicker for us to take her up than wait for them to come down and get her. It is much better for her to be there. They can start running some tests right away and she can go from there for her CT scan which is booked within the hour.

I have to admit, ICU is one of my least favourite places in the hospital. I'm not sure if it's the quiet I can't bear, broken only by the beeping instruments and the bellows-like sound of mechanical breathing. Maybe it's the lack of movement. No one ever really appears to be in a hurry in ICU. They all creep around in rubber-soled shoes, like a legion of Stepford nurses, no one ever breaking into a run. Stability is the name of the game here, and all they are ever doing is topping up drips or emptying IV bags, keeping people comfortable. The patients themselves don't move much. Most are in a coma, supposedly undergoing some sort of neurological rehab, which seems to involve just lying there while one relative after another sits by the bedside and hopefully squeezes their lifeless hand. Or they are simply deeply sedated as they recover from traumatic accidents or operations. I find the place incredibly depressing.

It really is God's waiting room. It is the last resort, where surgeons send their chronically ill patients in order not to have to deal with their hysterical relatives themselves. Rather than fessing up and admitting that the situation is totally hopeless, that the patient is brain-dead and unlikely ever to recover, they chicken out and pretend there is a chink of light at the end of a very long and very dark tunnel, and that if only their father, mother or son were to spend some time in ICU they might stand a chance. It's the coward's way out – passing the buck.

Another thing about ICU is that the relatives always expect miracles. They've seen so many TV shows where people suddenly wake up, have a stretch and a yawn, and the person at the bedside says something along the lines of 'Hello, Mum, what took you so long?', that they expect it to happen to them. When in fact it is hard work surviving ICU. You have to be fit. You have to be able to withstand the tubes, the drugs, the muscle-wasting, the inertia. It is difficult for the body to get through something so traumatic. If you were in bad shape before you went in, chances are you are not coming out alive. Only about 5 per cent of cardiac patients walk out of ICU. Actually, only about 10 per cent of patients survive a cardiac arrest full stop, but because of *Casualty* and *ER* people expect the majority of cardiac patients to 'pull through' in the end.

Doctors have also been known to lie to the consultants who run ICU and tell them their patient had a wonderful quality of life before going into ICU, so as to get them a bed. I remember Chris spinning some sort of yarn about an elderly woman a few months back, telling them she'd been up and about, walking to the shops, etc., when in fact she was a bedridden alcoholic whose daughter, visiting her once a day, kept her in sauce. The old biddy had fallen out of bed because she was so sozzled and landed on her head. Amazingly, she did leave the ICU standing on her own two feet, rather than feet first. So maybe Chris was right to lie.

One other thing that is shocking about ICU is the money it sucks in. Each bed costs about £1,800 a day to maintain and is surrounded by around £60,000 of equipment, and there's a nurse-to-bed ratio of one to one, which means that more often than not, due to the flexibility of numbers on the ward, they use agency nurses who cost on average four times more than the staff. Our ICU ward costs about £25,000 a day to keep open and just over £11.3 million a year. That is extremely expensive, but also, obviously, essential. Last year we had over three hundred operations cancelled at the last minute due to lack of intensive care beds, which of course entails an additional cost that has to be picked up elsewhere within the system.

We are met out of the lift by the head consultant of ICU. Her name is Jane McRae, and she is notoriously one of the most unpleasant people in the entire hospital. If she has not made a grown man cry by the end of the day, then that day is a disappointment to her.

'Morning,' she says, her dry mouth cracking into a coffee-stained smile. 'This our lady?'

'Yes,' says Margaret, as we both push the trolley along with its various IV stands and monitors. 'Her name is Rebecca Benson, she is thirty-four years old, and she has had a bump on the head—'

'Downtime uncertain,' I add. 'She's had CPR and we have given her—'

'We'll take it from here, dear,' says Ms McRae, tapping the back of my hand, in a manner that implies neither of us is worthy of crossing her threshold. 'Germs,' she adds, looking us both up and down.

I'm not sure if it is by way of description rather than explanation.

'Oh, right, fine,' I say. 'I'll direct her family up here, then, shall I?'

'That would be the simplest thing to do,' she replies.

I look her up and down in her pale yellow scrubs, with matching cap and shoe covers. It is hard to be patronizing looking like a great big lemon, but somehow she seems to manage it. It takes effort to harbour that much hatred for the human race. It can't be doing her much good.

'Jesus,' says Margaret as we get back in the lift, 'that woman is unpleasant.'

'Yup,' I agree.

'She's a jumped-up anaesthetist who hasn't had a fuck in years,' she adds, looking down and flicking fluff off her bosom.

Her hair is no longer shiny; it is covered in a dull crisp layer of hardened sperm. You have to admire her willingness to get on and down with it this early in the morning. Then again, there's nothing like seeing the daily results of the fickle hand of fate to make you grab that day-blow-job opportunity just a bit more firmly.

'D'you know which hospital Steve is going to tomorrow?' I ask as we watch the lift light descend through the floors.

'No,' she replies, looking at me like I need certifying.

'I just thought that—'

'I'd care? Or give a shit?' She smiles. 'Don't be ridiculous! How long have you worked here?'

'So you're not going . . . ?'

'Going out with him?' she shrieks. 'Since when?'

'I thought it might be a new thing.'

'A, I think Steve is seeing a Max Fox on the third floor. B, he is leaving tomorrow, so who cares? And C, I am too busy for a boyfriend.'

The lift pings. The doors open, and Margaret does a little indignant head wobble as she marches out of the lift.

'I was only asking!' I shout after her.

She turns around and gives me the finger.

I had no idea she liked him that much.

I just manage to get out of the lift myself before the lunch trolley crashes in. I look down at the stack of municipal green plates piled with peas, sweetcorn and non-specific meat stew and potatoes, each one covered with a transparent plastic lid. I check my watch. Who wants to eat lunch at 11.14 in the morning? And who wants to eat *that*? The food in this hospital is always bad and always turns up at the wrong time. The NHS shells out over

£500 million a year on food with a budget of £1.70 per person per day, which is for two meals, lunch and dinner; breakfasts and cups of tea come out of another budget. It doesn't sound a huge amount, 85p a meal, and when you realize that only 60 per cent of that is actually spent on food with the other 40 per cent going on overheads, you realize why the stuff looks so unpalatable. They get more money in the prisons, apparently, which doesn't seem right to me. We also don't have enough staff to serve the food, so instead of it taking a gang of twenty half an hour to get around the wards in this building they have four on the job and it takes anything between one and two hours. So what starts out as piping hot and, I suppose, edible becomes cold and inedible by the time it reaches the majority of patients, which obviously defeats the point. The ill are supposed to eat well, otherwise they will not improve. Looking at this crap, it almost makes you want to be HIV positive and in the Chelsea and Westminster, which reputedly has the best food in any hospital in the UK. Elton John pays for it. Or at least his foundation does. He does an extraordinary amount for HIV patients on the NHS. He pays for wings, dolls up existing wards and makes their lives a whole lot more pleasant.

I look at the shelf below the plates and retch slightly. I'm not sure if it's my hangover or if the sight of the congealed custard is enough to turn any man's stomach. It's rank. No wonder half the stuff comes back uneaten. And you get supper at 4.30 p.m., so once you've refused that there's nothing to keep you going till your cup of tea, roll and warm yoghurt in the morning.

'Don't worry,' says Louise as she walks past, 'they'll grow back.'

'What will?'

'Your bollocks,' she says, with a smile. 'I presume she ripped them off?'

'She is a total bitch.'

'We're cluttering up her ward. We've given her two patients today already.'

'Who else has gone up there?' I ask.

'The burns man. He was far too ill to sit down here waiting for plastics to turn up. He went up about half an hour ago.'

We both go over to the computer to get our next patient.

'Ladies first,' I say, gesturing towards the desk.

'Thanks, mate,' says Steve, barging in front. 'I need to get my stats up a bit.' He peers over the list. 'Any doctor referrals?' he sniffs. 'Aha. A nice urinary tract infection. Fingers crossed she's twenty-three!' He taps away on the screen.

Louise is next, taking an ankle sprain. 'Which leaves you with . . . oh, Mrs Singh and chest pain!' She smiles at me and I start to shake my head. This is going to be very annoying indeed.

'Mrs Singh?' I say, poking my head into the waiting room, which is now almost completely full.

The old ladies' tea party is in full swing in the corner as they munch on their biscuits and hang on Phillip Schofield's every word. He appears to be sharing with them next season's latest fashions, along with tips on how to mix and match trends. They all look gripped. Over in the far corner there's a mother and her son. He has a nosebleed but is undeterred as he holds his nose with one hand and tries to play his DS with the other. A few rows have been taken over completely by patients who have entirely given up the ghost. They are no longer listening out for their name and have passed out over the red plastic bucket seats, dead to the world.

'Mrs Singh?' I repeat, looking around the room, only to have my worst fears confirmed.

Mrs Singh is a large elderly lady of Indian origin and she is walking towards me with a sizeable family entourage comprising a son and daughter-in-law and three grandchildren, one a mewling and spewing babe in arms.

'Mrs Singh,' I smile. My teeth gritted.

The old woman nods.

'How is the chest?'

Mrs Singh grabs her rather ample right bosom and does her best to look pained. Meanwhile her granddaughter is talking about 'paining, paining, lots of paining'. I nod away, wanting to tell Mrs Singh that if she really wanted me to think that she might possibly have a heart condition, no matter how benign, she would at least get the correct bloody tit. Obviously I don't say that. I carry on smiling and usher the whole lot of them into a cubicle.

Mrs Singh is what is known in the trade as a 'health tourist'. She doesn't live in the UK, she does not pay UK taxes, but since she is visiting her son here in the UK who does pay UK taxes she has decided to take advantage of the NHS's free-at-the-point-of-demand policy and get herself a medical. When I worked in Ealing hospital for six months this time last year, health tourism used to drive us mad. It happens more in the summer and around Christmas, which is when families travel from the Indian subcontinent to see each other. And there is

nothing you can do about it, as you don't want to be the one
doctor who failed to spot a genuine case of angina because he
was trying to get an old biddy in and out of the hospital system
as quickly as possible. But I have to say, I really don't need Mrs
Singh and her entourage today. I am tired and, I think, rather
upset by Rebecca Benson. They always say that it's the
patients who are like you or who look like you or one of your
relatives who are the ones that affect you most, and I suppose
she is around my age. A little bit older, but even so, a con-
temporary of sorts. So what I don't need is a woman ligging a
freebie off the NHS, even if she is perfectly charming and in her
seventies. I quickly listen to her heart just to make sure she isn't
about to keel over on me, then walk out of the cubicle and pull
rank. Ewan is two years more junior than me and he doesn't
look busy, so I usher him in on the pretext that I might want
to show or teach him something. Not technically my job, grant
you, but Chris is busy and Ewan has made the mistake of
walking by. Before he quite realizes what has happened, even
as he is pumping up the blood pressure cuff, I am off and out
of there and clicking on my next patient.

My next is an ambulance delivery, which seems rather odd
for a young woman who appears to be perfectly capable of
walking and talking and indeed taking the bus.

'So' – I glance down to check her name – 'Jackie, what can
we do for you today?'

Dressed head to toe in pink velour, she is eighteen years old
and presenting with a headache.

'Well,' she says, running her hands through her very
dry, very white-blonde hair. She appears to have a ring

on every finger, as well as her thumb. 'I've got this headache.'

'Right.' I nod. 'Does it hurt when you look at bright lights?'

'Yes. Well, no. Well, a bit.'

'OK.' I nod again, and shine a torch into her pupils. She doesn't look away. Perhaps not meningitis then, I think. 'Do you have a rash anywhere?'

'No,' she coughs.

'Pains at the back of the neck? Do this.' I show her, putting my chin on my chest. She copies me. Not meningitis. 'Any other symptoms?'

'I am feeling sick,' she says.

'Have you been sick?'

'No. But I don't feel well. And I'm tired.' She yawns in my face. Her breath smells of old booze.

'Did you drink alcohol last night?'

'Yeah,' she says.

'How much?'

'Four White Lightning and half a bottle of cherry Lambrini,' she replies. 'Well, actually, nearly a bottle.'

'And you feel sick and you have a headache?' I can feel my pulse quickening and my palms beginning to sweat. I can feel the anger mounting. 'Do you possibly think that you might just have a hangover?'

'Yeah, maybe,' she shrugs.

'And you called an ambulance for a hangover?' I am beginning to raise my voice.

'Yeah, I might of,' she says. She is looking me in the eye. She doesn't seem ashamed or embarrassed. 'I'm entitled.'

'You are not entitled to a bloody ambulance to take you to hospital because you have a hangover.'

'What's going on in here?' asks Andrea, bustling in bosom first.

'Do you know how much an ambulance costs?' I continue, ignoring her. 'Eight hundred pounds.'

'Well, that's not my fault, is it!' she yells back at me, getting off her chair and putting her hands on her hips. 'This place is shit! You're all wankers! I don't need your help anyway!' And she marches off down the corridor like some pissed-off chat show contestant.

'Well we—' I start to yell after her.

'Don't,' says Andrea, putting her hand on my mouth. 'Stop. Breathe. And let it go. Otherwise you will be the one in trouble.'

She's right, I know. I'd be the one at a disciplinary hearing and she'd get to wag her many-ringed fingers at me while I watched my career go down the pan. I recall the surgeon and his extra croutons in the canteen. Shouting at patients is surely more of an offence than taking a few extra fried bread squares. I inhale and exhale and look up to see what I immediately fear is Rebecca Benson's husband sitting in tears in a chair clutching his toddler son. Chris Williams has a comforting hand on his shoulder.

'Come on,' says Andrea, following my gaze. 'There's a young woman in here who needs your help.'

She ushers me next door where the young woman in question is lying on the bed looking slightly terrified. Actually, now I look more closely, she is more of a child: she is wearing knee-length socks, a long pink skirt and a white T-shirt.

'This is Marsha,' Andrea announces. 'She is fifteen and has heavy pelvic bleeding.'

'Right,' I say, giving Marsha a smile.

She is quite a big girl, clearly fond of her grub, and she looks like she's in a bit of pain.

'Mum's just up the corridor, getting a coffee,' says Andrea, handing me a pair of surgical gloves.

'OK, then,' I nod. 'How long ago did the bleeding start, Marsha?'

'This morning,' she replies.

'Is it heavy?'

'And painful.'

'I'm just going to give you a quick pelvic examination. Would you mind removing your underwear?'

Marsha takes off her pants. There is a significant amount of blood and the girl does look quite uncomfortable. I put my hands up between her legs and straight away I can feel something hard and round. What the fuck is that? I lift up her skirt to take a closer look.

'Marsha?' I ask.

'Mmm?'

'Do you feel the urge to push?'

'Yes,' she replies.

'Yes, well, you're having a baby.'

'A baby?' her mother screams behind me, dropping two hot cups of coffee on the floor. 'A baby? You never told me you were pregnant!'

'I didn't know!' Marsha yells back.

'A baby?' The woman looks exasperated. 'You're only fifteen!'

All hell then breaks loose. Marsha is screaming with pain. Her mother is screaming with fury. I am screaming on the phone to get a midwife down from the second floor. I have delivered a baby or two but it was right at the beginning of my training and I didn't enjoy it very much. Also, Marsha is fifteen and has never been to an antenatal class in her life. The last thing she needs is another relative amateur at the business end telling her what to do.

Marsha is not that unusual. We usually get two or three girls in a year who give birth in A&E not knowing they were pregnant. They are usually young and usually Catholic and have said nothing for nine months because they were either terrified or in denial. Although Marsha does seem a little different in that she genuinely appears not to have known.

By the time a red-headed midwife called Mary arrives, some five minutes later, Marsha's mother, Denise, is sitting down in a chair in tears. 'No one knew, no one knew!' she keeps saying over and over again. 'And she's only fifteen!'

'Hello there,' says Mary, introducing a calm note to the fraught atmosphere. 'I am Mary and I am here to deliver the baby. Now, Mum' – she says this to Denise – 'you need to go up that end and hold . . .'

'Marsha,' I say.

'Hold Marsha's hand, because she is going to need some help to push this baby out.' She smiles, and turns to me. 'And you, you need to give me a hand. How dilated is she? What is her blood pressure? Can we get our hands on a foetal heart monitor?'

We both look at Marsha. She's a big girl, never mind that she's full term. Neither of us is sure the foetal heart monitor is going to be any use.

Obesity is a huge problem for the NHS. Fat people are more difficult to move and operate on, they are more likely to fall ill, they heal more slowly and they are more likely to have complications such as diabetes. The big problem, excuse the pun, in Maternity is you can't hear a tiny heartbeat through all the flesh. It is essential to hear the baby's heart during the birth process because there is no other way of determining if the baby is in distress or pain, or needs to come out right away. Therefore anyone with a body mass index over 40 uses up extra staff, as someone has to hold the foetal heart monitor hard against the flesh so that the midwife or consultant stands a chance of hearing it. The heart monitor holders are usually medical students and they can be made to stand there for up to twelve hours at a time. Obese mothers-to-be are also the anaesthetist's nightmare. Can you imagine how hard it is to anaesthetize a large woman in labour? It's enough to make them go for two big syringes at once!

Marsha utters an enormous low moan that grows into another scream.

'OK,' says Mary, crouching low between Marsha's legs. 'There's no time for anything. This baby's coming into the world whether we are ready or not. Marsha, listen to me. I am going to ask you to push, and when I tell you to stop pushing, you stop. OK?'

A strained 'OK' is all that Marsha can manage.

'OK now, push!' commands Mary. 'Like it's coming out of your bottom!'

'Push, baby, push!' Denise joins in.

'Push!' I find myself saying.

Marsha's entire face turns bright red and she lets out an enormous scream.

'That's it!' says Mary. 'Now stop! We have the head!' Mary runs her fingers quickly around the head to check for the umbilical cord. 'OK, my Marsha, just two more big pushes. Two . . . big . . . pushes. Push!'

'Aaaarrrrrrrgh!' screams Marsha.

'Oh my God!' screams her mother.

'It's a girl!' declares Mary as a fat, grey squirming thing slithers out on to the trolley. It opens its small toothless mouth and yells. 'Well done, Marsha. You have what looks like a very healthy little girl.'

12–1 p.m.

I'm not even halfway through my shift and I'm already shattered and in my second pair of scrubs for the day. I'm quite relieved when Mary asks if I'd like to come outside and have a cigarette. Perhaps not the healthiest example to patients, I admit. We're always preaching that patients should give up smoking if they are to get an operation on the NHS, which is obviously rich coming from a staff at least half of whom smoke. But hypocrisy was ever thus.

'You guys need to learn to deliver babies a bit better,' says Mary, leaning against the redbrick wall of the hospital and taking a long deep drag on her cigarette. 'It's pathetic the way you all come running to us as soon as you see a screaming fat woman.'

Short and stocky with her henna-dyed bob, Mary is one of the younger midwives so is on a twelve-and-a-half-hour shift for which she will be paid about £38,000 a year. But her rise through the ranks and up the pay band scale will be fast. Before, time served was an indicator of how much you'd be paid, now, if you have a degree you will earn more money more quickly. Her contract will, however, be a little more rigorous than those of the older midwives who have, over the years, managed to negotiate two days, day shifts only or weekend jobs as they have families of their own. She can already earn significant overtime, which can easily take her to £50,000 a year, but then she has plenty of responsibility. She used to specialize in drug-addicted pregnancies but has recently moved on to teenage pregnancies. Needless to say, we see a fair number of them in A&E.

'Thing is,' I say, after taking such a deep drag on my fag that I've given myself a bit of a head rush, 'I'm not that keen on the whole birth thing. It stinks for a start.'

'Don't breathe in,' she replies. 'Anyway, we all know that you doctors would much prefer it if the mothers had a simple C-section and a whole load of drugs.'

'I like those TOBP women. I can appreciate why they are tired of being pregnant and want a C-section and then a nice lunch. It makes it quieter and easier, that's for sure.'

'D'you know,' says Mary, flicking ash at her feet, 'you can always tell a smoker by their grey, gritty placenta.'

'I think I saw pictures of that when I was training,' I say. 'That and the gonorrhoea baby covered in gunk. Its eyes stuck shut . . . I actually now want to be sick.'

'Even I haven't seen one of those, and I've seen pretty much everything,' she says. 'Crack babies, smack babies, babies so small they fit entirely in one hand.'

It must be quite depressing running a unit looking after the youngest addicts in town and having to watching them shiver and vomit their way through withdrawal. Quite a few of the drug-dependent pregnancies are women off the streets. Either that or they have been living in hostels or bedsits. There is usually a multi-discipline team on hand after the baby is born to see if the child needs to be taken into care. They hang around to see if the mother bonds with the baby, doesn't leave it crying, and to assess whether she's suffering from post-natal depression and might self-harm.

'Wasn't she young,' I remark, thinking of Marsha and her incredibly shocked mother.

'Young?' replies Mary. 'I had a girl of twelve in last week.'

'Twelve?'

'Yup. You know, one of those lost girls in the care system who gets pregnant because there's nothing else to do and because school isn't for them.'

'Only to repeat the whole cycle all over again,' I sigh.

'Teenage mums are nearly always daughters of teenage mums,' Mary agrees. 'We had four generations in the other day. She was fourteen, her mum was thirty, I think, *her* mum was late forties, and *her* mum was in her sixties. Extraordinary. They all seemed quite happy about it. It was a very nice little baby.'

'Who was the father?'

'Oh, some fifteen-year-old toe-rag.'

'I don't suppose that was a water birth with twenty scented candles and a whole load of om shanti,' I say, stubbing my fag out on the ground.

'God,' Mary says. 'Really, never do one of those. I had a posh woman in the other day who'd had the whole water birth thing set up in her sitting room. You know, the paddling pool and candles, all in a bay window. The midwife was on her way when the contractions really kicked off. The woman pushed out a poo and the husband panicked and ran around trying to fish the thing out with a net. He then slipped over in the poo water and the candles fell off the pool and set fire to the curtains. Meanwhile the woman was screaming, giving birth. The husband eventually had to call the fire brigade and the woman actually gave birth in the ambulance in the street. And,' she adds with a smile, 'there's nothing om shanti about that!'

'Christ!' I laugh.

'Moral of that story?' she asks.

'Don't shit in the birthing pool?'

'Don't have a birth plan,' she says, flicking her fag butt across the car park. 'Shall we go?'

I follow Mary back into the hospital through the side door. We are both chewing a mint like a couple of teenagers trying not to be caught smoking.

'See you later,' she says. 'We'll take good care of Marsha.'

I pause and take a breath, bracing myself before going back into A&E. It's only when I slip through the swing doors that I realize something major has gone down while I've been flicking fag ash on the pavement round the back. There are police everywhere. Not your usual gentle bobby with a pen and pencil and an old granny who's had a dizzy spell at the bus stop. Armed police. SO19. They've got their semi-automatic machine guns out, their flak jackets on, and they are crawling all over the place.

Andrea rushes past, her white plastic apron covered in blood, in her hands a stainless-steel tray full of bloody swabs. 'Where the fuck have you been?' she barks at me, exuding professionalism. 'Didn't you get your page?'

'Page?'

'Yes, your fucking page.'

I rather sheepishly pull my pager out of my scrubs trouser pocket. It's switched off. I almost begin to explain that I haven't left A&E all shift and I was just taking some air after delivering a baby, but I can see that she does not give a flying fuck what weedy excuse I have.

'Get yourself in there with Steve,' she tells me, flicking her head in the direction of the closest resus bay. 'We've got three with severe gunshot wounds. Some gangland shoot-out.'

Oh fuck, I think as I snap on some fresh gloves and pull back the curtains, there's no time to scrub in for this. We need to stabilize this bloke right now and it's going to be messy.

The problem with firearms injuries in this country is that half the villains don't know how to shoot. They use the wrong weapons, with the wrong ammunition, which doesn't kill you, so you don't get a nice clean bullet hole, a nice clean shot, or indeed a nice clean death. It is always such a bloody mess.

We had a bloke in the other day who was either incredibly stupid or incredibly unlucky, I never quite worked out which. Either way, he stole a car that was full of drugs. It had something like a million pounds' worth of cocaine in it, which he drove off with, much to the irritation and annoyance of the gangs involved. Obviously the said gangs wanted their car and coke back so they shot him twelve times, nine times in the back as he was running away. He only survived because none of them could shoot properly, but the mess was terrible. They shattered his shoulder blade, ribs and arms; he lost the right one completely, we just couldn't put it back together. He did, incredibly, manage to walk out of here about three weeks later.

But this guy might take a little longer than that. Steve's already cracked his chest and opened him up like a cadaver in an anatomy class, he's wired up to a heart monitor, he's being given pure oxygen, and there are three empty bags of O neg on the side.

'Good to see you,' says Steve, amazingly without a hint of sarcasm. 'I can't find this fucking bullet, there's too much blood. Can you give us a hand?'

For a bloke who's about to bugger off up north and specialize in kids, Steve has done his fair share of bullet holes. Before coming here he spent six months in east London just when there was a turf war between the Yardies and the Turks as the Russians moved in – or some such unsavoury Euro melange. Anyway, they had bodies coming in on a regular basis; he used to joke that it was like doing a tour as a medic in Vietnam. Although even Louise, I remember her saying, had two shootings and four stabbings, one through the heart, when she was in sleepy Eastbourne – something to do with rival Lithuanian gangs. It seems nowhere is immune these days.

I step in and start suctioning around in the man's chest while Steve fishes through his lacerated flesh and punctured organs. The man, who looks Eastern European, is so pumped full of drugs he is dead to the world. I look over to see Andy sitting on his gas canisters, fumbling between his big syringe and his little syringe; he has beads of sweat glistening on his fat top lip. He catches my eye, but appears to look straight through me. The beeps on the heart monitor start to slow down.

'Pressure's dropping,' Andy says, stating the obvious.

There's always a bit of a battle between the surgeon and the anaesthetist when it comes to an operation, but this sort in particular. The doctor likes the blood pressure to be nice and low so as to minimize the bleeding, and the anaesthetist likes the pressure high as it means the blood and brain are oxygenating properly.

'Thanks, Andy,' says Steve, somewhat tersely. 'We all have ears.'

'I was just saying,' he replies.

'Can you see anything?' Steve asks me, huffing through his mask.

'D'you want me to have a go?' I ask.

'Go on,' he says, stepping aside.

I hand over the suction tube, he gives me the tweezers, and I start searching.

'I've taken two bullets out already,' he continues, indicating a small metal dish containing two bloodied slugs. 'There's another in the arm, above that snake tattoo.' He points. 'And there's another in here, but I'm damned if I can find it.'

We both lean over. The man's insides are all red and shiny and gelatinous, like a shaken-up Christmas trifle. I follow the direction of Steve's tube, peering in where he has cleared the blood.

'Shall I go and get some more blood?' asks one of the Filipina nurses, whose name I am ashamed to say I don't know.

'That would be good,' says Steve, without looking up. 'Just in case we don't get the bastard soon.'

'There!' I say, stopping the nurse in her tracks. I gently move a piece of flesh. 'Just behind the liver. He's a lucky boy, it just clipped the bottom as it went in.'

'Well, not that lucky,' says Steve.

'I imagine a good shooting is an occupational hazard in his line of work,' I say. 'What did he do anyway?' I'm slowly taking the bullet out while trying not to damage any other organs as I do so.

'Guns or drugs,' says Steve, 'something like that. I wasn't really listening when the police were telling me, I was much more interested in cutting his shirt off. All I know is that it was two against one, and he was the one, although he seems to have given them a healthy run for their money.'

'Who's with the others?'

'Chris, Louise and Ewan, and I think, thankfully, Ian came in early.'

Ian is another A&E consultant who is just that bit less senior than Chris but who is also extremely good at his job, despite his fondness for poppers and clubs at the weekend. He is good-looking and very popular with the staff, mainly because he's always got an opinion, a joke and a filthy story. He is the perfect person to sympathize with your hangover. Although last night he was not his usual badly behaved self. For a start, he did not hog the karaoke like he did at Christmas, when he finished the evening crashed out among the spinning beer bottles and streamers. Perhaps he's grown up, got his eye on a senior consultancy, and is trying to set an example to the juniors.

The bullet clatters into the metal tray and both Steve's and my shoulders move a few centimetres away from our ears. What a relief. There is nothing worse than searching through someone's insides trying to find a bullet. The pressure mounts and the longer you take the less positive the prognosis gets. And you can't really leave it in there. Some people live happily for years with bullets and shrapnel lodged in their flesh, but it is not an ideal scenario.

It takes Steve and me another twenty minutes or so to locate the other bullet in his arm and stitch him up. Sadly, neither of us is at that top surgeon stage where the patients are made ready for us – anaesthetized, laid out and opened – awaiting our crucial incisions, only for us to leave immediately after, our rarefied hands held slightly in the air, as someone else does the closing and finishes and clears up around us. It is no wonder really, with that sort of service, that most top surgeons are arrogant arses with terrible God complexes who find it hard to relate to their patients as anything more than a bit of flesh surrounded by green material. They are no longer patients with problems, they are just a problem, or indeed in some cases just a nameless tumour. Although obviously I too am looking forward to the day when I can become an arrogant arse, as there is nothing more boring than stitching up. There are also some people you make a bit more of an effort with. I am much more likely to try to get the scar all neat and small and compact if the patient is a young woman who has been in a car accident rather than, say, some tattooed gangster who's blown ten tons of shit out of a few work colleagues.

Louise, Chris and Ian are still with their patients when Steve and I come out. The police are looking particularly grim-faced as they ask us for the bullets, to be bagged as evidence. From talking to them, it sounds like one of the other blokes is touch and go at the moment, so our bloke may well wake up to find that not only does he look like a patchwork quilt, he's also going to be charged with murder.

'Has he said anything?' one copper asks me.

'He was out cold and intubated by the time I saw him,' I reply.

'And how many bullets?'

'Four.'

I walk back up the corridor towards the common room. I have definitely earned myself a full fat Coke break, I think, and, looking down at my blood-spattered scrubs, another change of clothes.

Freshly kitted out in my third pair of scrubs, I make my way into the common room. The place is packed with nurses eating their lunches, all brought in from home. They sit together, huddled in groups that are very much divided along racial lines. There are the Filipinas in one corner, many of them tucking into plastic containers of rice or noodles with the occasional fish head thrown in, while over in another corner is the African contingent, some munching on sandwiches, others digging into their rice and yams with a little lamb or goat garnish. And never the twain shall meet. In fact, there is practically a form of apartheid that goes on among the nursing staff, with the remaining Brits and Irish as a buffer zone. It's not that they hate each other, they are just much happier working in their different gangs. They will work together if they have to, but they would rather not.

The nursing community has changed very much in the last few years. The days of finding the likes of Abi Titmuss in her push-up bra and stay-up stockings emptying your bedpan are over. Nowadays the nurses, particularly in the capital or in the inner-city hospitals, are almost entirely Filipina or African. In fact, if it weren't for Filipina nurses the NHS would grind to a halt. After the Irish went back to Ireland when they realized they could earn just as much money at home, the NHS decided it had to recruit elsewhere. Some drives, like the ones in the Philippines, were successful; others, like the one in West Africa, went spectacularly wrong.

A few years back, the NHS recruited a group of nurses from Nigeria to work in the UK. However, when they arrived in this country it turned out that 60 per cent of them were HIV positive. So, instead of working for the NHS, they became patients. There is a rule that if you come to this country and you are HIV positive, you have an automatic right to stay. It is one of your many human rights. There was a huge amount of HIV tourism to the UK in the early nineties, people arriving and then declaring that they had the virus, which meant that they could not be sent home. Oddly, this seems to have slowed down of late due to the fact that we no longer fund ongoing HIV treatment here in the UK and HIV treatment in Africa is now a little better.

So the likes of Margaret and Andrea are the last of a dying

breed. And as a result, the sexual politics of the wards have also changed. Nigerian and Filipina nurses tend not to put out that much. So sadly there are not so many doctors-and-nurses games any more. Randy, drunk student doctors have had to find other prey to sex-pest. They more usually have their sights set on the growing number of randy, drunk student female doctors, or indeed the physios. You usually need straight As at A-level to become a physio and they tend to be quite a sporty bunch of bright, sparky girls, which is the sort of criteria that suits an over-sexed student doctor down to the ground.

The African/Filipina stand-off continues in food-chomping silence. Occasionally there's some inter-group dialogue, in a dialect that only three people in the room can understand, but otherwise the atmosphere of mutual mistrust is broken only by the smell of exotic food, which is gently overtaking the room. I'm leafing through the pages of a rubbish celebrity magazine and waiting for the kettle in the corner to boil.

Ian walks in and looks over my shoulder. 'Botox . . . Botox . . . Botox . . . fillers . . . Sculptra . . . Fuck me! Look at the trout pout on that!' he declares as his very clean, very manicured finger jabs its way along a line of orange-coloured bridesmaids at some celeb nuptials. 'And the whole bloody lot of them have been Tangoed! Some massive napalm bomb of fake tan has been sprayed all over the wedding. Jesus Christ, is that the dad?' He squints in closer for another look.

'How's your gangster?' I ask.

'He lives! It was like raising Lazarus, though. We nearly lost him twice. But so good to know that he has been saved and can now murder and traffic drugs again, don't you think?'

The kettle flicks off.

'Coffee?'

'No thanks,' he says. 'I just came in to see what I can steal from the fridge. I am bloody starving and the drugs lunch isn't for another half-hour. Are you going?'

'Free sandwiches,' I reply. 'What's not to love?'

'How's your head from last night?'

'Bad. Yours?'

'Quite shit,' he admits. 'I hate cheap alcohol. Note to self: stop drinking wine out of a box. But you know what they say. Nothing like a good gang shoot-out to clear the cobwebs!' He opens the fridge and looks over the shelves and in the door. 'Oh God,' he sighs. 'Where's a wrapped KitKat when you need one?'

'Hi there,' says a very clean-shaved, keen-faced bloke as he pokes his head round the door. 'David. Plastics? I'm looking for Mr Williams.'

'Ah,' says Ian, checking him over with a swift expert glance. 'He's just saving the life of a terribly nice gangster. Can we help?'

'I was wondering why the place was crawling with SO19.' David smiles.

'This is a charming neighbourhood,' observes Ian.

'I think he wanted you to look at our burns man,' I say.

'Right,' he nods. 'Accident, assault or self-immolation?'

'He set fire to himself in Sainsbury's car park.'

'Oh dear,' says David. 'That's sad.'

'He's forty-five per cent, and I think he's in ICU.' I take a sip of my coffee. He watches me intently. 'Um, do you want a cup before you go up and see him?'

'Oh no,' he says, his face scrunching up in disgust. 'I know my tremor triggers,' he adds, holding out the most immaculately maintained pair of hands I have ever seen.

Plastic surgeons tend to be a little obsessive. It is one of the most competitive disciplines to get into, and therefore attracts the highest achievers from medical school. As their job requires an eye for detail and concentrated patience, this often translates into pernickety and mannered behaviour outside the operating theatre. When I was in Bognor we used to have a visiting plastics bloke who refused to carry his own box of instruments in case he injured himself. He would arrive like the star turn and demand that two orderlies help with £15K worth of kit, always claiming that his hands were his tools and he didn't want to damage or strain them with heavy work of any kind. Needless to say, the rest of us weren't exactly enamoured with him.

'Let me take you up there,' I say to David, turning around to pour my coffee down the sink.

'Tremor triggers,' I hear Ian spit, under his breath. 'Just put your elbows on the fucking table.'

1–2 p.m.

Having deposited David and his £1,300 custom-made surgical magnifying specs that he got from the States in the ICU with the harridan McRae, I make a speedy exit down the stairs. I had no idea the lift journey from A&E up to ICU could take so long. I heard all about Dave's specs and his last three burns victims before thankfully we were forced apart by a bloke with a broken leg on his way back from X-ray.

Back down in A&E and there are still SO19 everywhere. It does rather change the atmosphere of a place to have armed police patrolling around, especially when you are supposed to be reaching out to your community.

'Are you coming to the drugs lunch?' asks Louise as she approaches in a fresh pair of scrubs.

'What are they selling?'

'I've no idea, I'm just after the free sarnies. M&S apparently.'

'Nice. I'm in.'

'Drugs lunch,' says Steve, tapping the side of his nose as he walks over to the computer. 'Starts in fifteen.'

'Absolutely,' says Louise. 'I am bloody starving. Some bastard stole my KitKat from the fridge!'

'Terrible,' I say, hoping my cheeks are not as red as they feel.

Once a week, or twice a month, or whenever anyone can get it together, we have what is known as In-House Teaching, which is when one of the surgeons or doctors comes in and shares a few pearls with us over what is laughably called our lunch break. Not to be confused with the Grand Round, which is very grand and round, when glamorous, important surgeons come and share their splendid knowledge with us, and half the hospital turns out to pay its respects. An In-House Teaching session is much more informal, more social, and obviously a whole lot less useful. But we do get to sit in rows and eat our lunch while listening to someone wang on about something they did last week. The idea is that they can still say we are being 'trained on the job' and are not working our guts out at the coalface of healthcare.

Occasionally, however, the In-House Teaching session is given over to a drugs company with some new pills to flog. They take over the hall and fill it full of leaflets and charts and, most importantly, sandwiches and doughnuts – and if we are extremely lucky, hot snacks – and we go and listen for half an hour and get fed for our generosity. Like the bunch of canapé mercenaries that we are: no one really cares what they are selling, just so long as we get some food. Most of the time the drugs rep is singing the praises of a drug we already use, which always seems a little pointless to me. Sometimes they extol the virtues of a drug we don't use, but seeing as none of us in the room has the power to purchase a new drug for the NHS, I also think this seems a little pointless. But they say they are networking us for the future. Planting seeds in our addled little brains so that when we are powerful, with corporate cheque-books in our briefcases, we'll come knocking on their door because they gave us a prawn sandwich and a bag of salt and vinegar crisps eight years back.

It is all rather doubtful, I think, especially as each hospital has its own drugs policy, which is dictated by NICE (the National Institute for Health and Clinical Excellence) and is fairly simple: we try to keep costs down and buy the cheapest drugs unless there is an important reason not to. But because the NHS orders in such vast quantities, it is a sitting duck for drugs companies who want to take advantage of the bulk ordering system, particularly if they have a monopoly on selling the drug in the first place.

In the last couple of years there have been some staggering price hikes for some of the most basic drugs. Flucloxacillin syrup, which is one of the most common antibiotics prescribed for children with throat infections etc., used to cost us £4 per 125ml bottle but has now gone up to over £20. The five-fold increase came about after one drugs company became the sole supplier of the syrup. The purchase of this drug alone will cost the taxpayer an extra £44 million a year. And they are not the only ones. Gabapentin, an anti-epilepsy drug, has gone up from £5.52 per 600mg to over £41. Cimetidine, a treatment for stomach ulcers, has risen from £16 per 800mg pack to over

£22. But perhaps the worst offenders are hydrocortisone tablets, of which the NHS buys sixty thousand packets a month: they have rocketed from £5 per 10g to £44.40. The company responsible is blaming a need for a new factory to make the pills, but it is we who are footing the bill. Let no one ever say that pharmaceutical companies are in the business out of the kindness of their own hearts! So I don't feel at all guilty about filling my pockets with pens and sandwiches, and sitting there trying to do the *Times* crossword while they witter on about statins.

I went to a statins dinner a couple of months back. The specialist trainee who is in charge of Grand Rounds and talks had managed to get the statins company to sponsor dinner in the Chinese around the corner. We had to listen to the talk about a statin we already prescribed in the hospital by the truckload for about twenty minutes, while shovelling in as much chow mein and free beer as we could. I have to say it got quite ugly after the rep left. Well, he made the mistake of leaving another £200 behind the bar, which we all thought was our duty to use up as quickly as possible. I made a bit of a tit of myself by telling Louise that I fancied her; she has been gracious enough never to mention it since. I am hoping, obviously, that she can't remember the incident. But somehow I know she can. She is the sort of ambitious, go-getting woman who always has total recall at the end of a night – mainly because she doesn't get completely plastered like the rest of us.

In olden days, though, drugs companies used to splash out a bit more than taking fifteen doctors to the Lotus Flower. I have a mate who just after he was made a consultant was flown to

South Africa, Hawaii and Rome, all first class, within a month. I'm not sure what they were hoping he might do for them, but they were very much on the charm offensive. Sadly, the drugs companies have recently decided to save themselves some cash and have signed up to the Association of the British Pharmaceutical Industry guidelines committing them to fly their doctors economy class, which is nowhere near as much fun and obviously takes the shine off any foreign trip.

But all the flights and entertainment do work. Some doctors get caught up in the drugs company whirl and find themselves pronouncing on the merits of such and such a drug. GPs are a little more susceptible because the ailments they're treating are usually not so life-threatening, so the merits of one drug over another are all much of a muchness. If you're a specialist it's a lot less witty to prescribe something because it reminds you of your recent trip to Florida. But that didn't stop a few doctors overzealously claiming extraordinary things. There was one who declared that he had found the cure for MS. He went from conference to conference announcing the miracle drug – forgetting to question the P-value, which is the statistical measure of something happening by chance. When the smoke disappeared from up his arse and the PR lunches dried up, he was left looking rather embarrassed.

The world of plastic surgery is a little more murky. There are obviously plenty of private clinics that are a lot less regulated than the NHS, and they are not governed by NICE, so they can take as many kickbacks and jolly weekends abroad as they like. I have a mate who does plastics for the NHS as well as working for a private clinic and he is full of stories of dodgy doctors recommending one type of filler over another because they've been slipped a little extra. There's one who lauded one filler at a meeting in Miami, only to be heard backing something else three months later at a conference in New York. He was being paid to do 'research' for the different drugs companies, which clearly consisted of him going from gathering to gathering telling everyone how marvellous their stuff was.

When drugs companies discovered the power of celebrity, no one needed creepy doctors selling their reputations for twelve holes in Palm Springs so much any more. Viagra sales were fairly moribund until Jack Nicholson was busted taking the drug back in 2001, when his then girlfriend Lara Flynn Boyle was pictured collecting his prescription at the chemist. One sniff of celeb endorsement and sales went through the roof. Jack then later proclaimed, 'I only take Viagra when I am with more than one woman.' Which of course sent sales up even further. Obviously, given the nature of the beast, there is a limit to the number of medical products that can attract a celebrity endorsement; no one is going to admit using Anusol pile cream because it helps them sit longer. Then again, Bill Clinton did up the sales of Siemens Signia hearing aids when he was pictured using one at an international conference.

'I hope the talk is better than the Jehovah's Witness we had last week,' says Steve, typing at the computer.

'I didn't go,' I say. 'I didn't fancy the idea of religious sandwiches.'

'Oh, the snacks were good,' he insists. 'Hummus and everything.'

'I can't stand a chickpea.'

'Really?' He looks up at me. 'One of my favourite things. I love a falafel, with pitta and sauce. God I'm hungry. How long till this lunch?'

'Excuse me,' Jon Berry chips in with his whining nasal tones, 'this is not an area for staff to use their communication skills.'

'What?' says Steve.

'This is not an area for vocalizing, communicating . . . talking. The communication area is the common room. This is a designated work area. For work.'

'Right,' says Steve, not looking at Jon, who is rocking back and forth on thick soles. 'Anyway, as I was saying, there is this great place near me – Falafel King. I am there every Saturday. Bloody delicious, it really is.'

'I think they taste like ear wax,' I say, reaching down and clicking on another patient.

'Ear wax? Do you eat ear wax?'

'How long has that one been waiting?' asks Jon, poking his spotty chin over my shoulder. 'Oh, three hours ten.'

'There's been a gang shooting,' says Steve, pointing to the two armed police pacing up and down the corridor.

'That's as may be,' Jon responds, 'but rules are rules.'

'Yes, well, she's in under four hours so everyone's happy,' I say.

'At three hours ten, *she* won't be,' says Steve.

And he's not wrong. Sarah Clark is so pissed off by the time I pull back the curtain to treat her that she can barely be bothered to look up from her iPhone.

'Some of us have got jobs,' she says. 'I have been sitting here all morning.'

'I am very sorry for the delay,' I say. 'We have had quite a large incident come into the hospital this morning.'

'Really,' she says, sounding unimpressed.

'That's why we have all the police here,' I add.

'Yeah, well. Back to me. I have a stomach ache and I think I've got appendicitis.'

'Really,' I say. 'OK, if you pop up on to the bed and let me take a look. How long has it been hurting?'

'Ever since I woke up this morning.'

'So, not too long then? Are you having your period at the moment?'

'No,' she answers. 'It's my appendix. It says here that the symptoms I've got are appendicitis.' She flashes her iPhone at me. '"Pain in the lower abdomen that after to four or five hours will localize." Well, I haven't been in pain for that long yet . . .'

If there's anything more annoying than a pissed-off patient, it's a pissed-off patient with access to Google. I have lost count of the number of times a patient has sat there and told me I am wrong, or that my diagnosis is incorrect. They are almost always young, with an iPhone in their hand, or they have printed a whole load of stuff off the internet before coming in. It's a generational thing. No one in their eighties would question a doctor's judgement. Yet someone who has no medical training whatsoever thinks it is perfectly fine to look you in the eye and say 'I've looked it up on the internet and you are completely wrong.' And then they start quoting stuff back at you that is invariably crap and invariably from the States, where the protocol is different and usually more cost-based. I had an argument only last week when I suggested to someone that they would have to stay in hospital another twenty-four hours after their operation for observation, and they started to shout at me that I was wrong, flashing some website results from a hospital in Baltimore. Also, of course, nowadays, due to all the press reports about cutbacks, everyone accuses you of trying to save money rather than doing something for the good of the patient. 'You're just doing that because it's cheaper,' they say. No one listens when you argue otherwise.

I start to feel around Ms Clark's stomach for anything swollen or out of the ordinary, while she continues to type away on her iPhone.

'On a scale of one to ten, how painful is it?' I ask.

'Ten, obviously,' she replies. 'Otherwise I wouldn't have sat in the waiting room for all this time, would I?'

'No, of course.'

I push in the middle of her stomach, which is quite taut and hard, ballooned even. I push again. Then she lets off an enormous loud long fart. I bite the inside of my cheek to stop myself from laughing.

'Better?' I ask, my voice slightly strained.

'I'm fine,' she says, swinging her legs swiftly off the bed and pulling down her shirt. She quickly picks up her handbag, her cheeks burning red. 'How the hell do you get out of this place?'

I follow her out of the bay and point her in the direction of the exit. I have never seen anyone move so fast. She doesn't turn back and she doesn't say thank you.

'That was quick,' says Steve.

'A bad case of wind,' I reply.

'Excellent,' he smirks. 'Shall we go and grab some lunch?'

When we get to the lecture hall, the place is packed. It's amazing how many staff will turn out for a free ham roll. There's a long table below the line of large sash windows on the other side of the room that is covered in plastic trays of party-pack sandwiches.

'Great,' says Steve, 'Marks and Spencer. Come on, we'd better get stuck in before it all goes.'

Steve and I grab a white plastic plate each and start to pile on as many sandwiches as we can. Then we find a pew far enough back so as not to have to engage in any way with the speaker, and start to scoff. I have a mouth full of egg and cress when Louise suddenly appears out of nowhere.

'Can I sit here?' she asks.

I can only mumble something vaguely positive-sounding, which she takes for a yes and sits down.

'Jesus,' she says, clocking my plate, 'don't hold back.'

'I'm hungry,' I mutter.

'I can see that,' she says, taking the corner off a prawn sandwich. 'Nice to see half the hospital here.'

She is exaggerating slightly, but the turnout is large. Each of the departments is more or less sitting together in their teams. The surgeons are sitting apart from the physicians and there is a healthy air of disrespect emanating from each of the groups. The cardiologists think they are better than the oncologists, the paediatricians think they are better than the orthopaedists, and everyone, obviously, thinks they are better than A&E. But what is more amusing is that the surgeons think they are better than the doctors and the doctors think that the surgeons are no better than Neanderthals and only one up from the barber-surgeons of the eighteenth century. Some of the doctors take great pleasure in addressing surgeons as Mr, just to remind them of a time when surgeons were tradesmen who were not properly trained. They really do think that they just walk into an operating theatre, saw off a leg while listening to Tina Turner's 'Simply the Best', and walk straight out again.

Sitting next to Louise, I am suddenly conscious that egg sandwiches were perhaps not the sexiest choice, as each time she leans in to talk to me all I can think of is the waft of eggy breath she must be getting with my reply.

'Good afternoon everyone!' begins the drugs rep, walking into the middle of the room.

I look between the shoulders of the paeds in front of me. 'Oh my God,' I say to Steve. 'She used to sit next to me in anatomy class. Her name is Karen.'

'My name is Karen,' says Karen, 'and I am here to talk to you about statins.'

'Really?' Steve says.

'Yeah. She was always quite weird. She used to keep her packed lunch inside her body.'

'What? The cadaver?'

'Yup,' I whisper. 'She'd pop her sandwiches in the heart cavity when the lecturer came round.'

'Gross,' says Steve.

I used to love anatomy class. Two years of total enjoyment. There is something quite amazing about being allowed to cut up someone's body and get right in there. It is also amazing that people actually leave their bodies to science in the first place. And they are mostly not old doctors, they are ordinary people who leave their bodies to the London Anatomy Office. Just so long as they don't die of cancer, or have certain pathologies that render them abnormal, we get to chop them up. Very respectfully, of course. Their organs are taken out and bagged and tagged, the body is preserved, and at the end of the year they are all put back together to make a complete corpse. We then go to a Service of Thanksgiving at Southwark Cathedral. It's an extraordinary event, a rather moving and well-attended service. The families of the dead come and celebrate along with the students. After a year you do get to know your body quite well, so it's an odd feeling to meet the family and find out who they were in real life. It is a most extraordinary day.

Although, sadly, things are a little different these days. Since 2004 there have been many more students to a body, up from four to twelve, and a lot of the time they come pre-dissected. It's all supposed to save money, as looking after these bodies is expensive, but it does mean that students have much less hands-on experience than they used to.

'I wonder why she became a drugs rep,' I whisper. 'She was actually quite good.'

'Oh, that's easy,' says Steve. 'She gets her own car, phone, and quite a lot of cash. Meanwhile, we have to scrabble around hoping for some spare egg sandwiches.'

'Mmm,' I say, biting into my fourth sandwich.

Karen carries on telling a room full of bored digesting doctors about the marvellousness of a drug they already prescribe while I try to work out how I might get Louise's telephone number by the end of my shift. Or is she really having an affair with Chris? I've only got four hours left in the place to find out. I had better get cracking.

2–3 p.m.

I stay behind for a few minutes after the talk to have a chat with Karen. All I learn is that she is really happy, doing really well, is really happily married, has a really nice baby, and is earning seven grand a year more than me and working half the bloody hours. So I am really glad I hung around to ask all those helpful questions. I did also witness Steve scrabbling around and pocketing three free pens, which somehow added to my feelings of underachieving inadequacy.

How can she be earning £7,000 more than me? I pace along the corridor towards the door. I really need a cigarette. I am on a basic of about £30K for a forty-hour week, and with over-time and the bit extra I get for working at the coalface of humanity I can usually get it up to about £42,000. And that's for getting shouted at, puked on and covered in blood for over ten hours a day. While she swans around in her Mini Cooper, chatting about statins and handing out free sandwiches.

Outside, I light my cigarette and lean against the redbrick wall.

'Back again?' comes a familiar voice.

'And you,' I say to Mary, who's halfway down her Consulate. 'All OK up there?'

'Not bad,' she says, fluffing up her red hair. 'Marsha has named her child Destiny.'

'OK,' I say. 'That was quick.'

'I know. Makes me wonder if she did know all along. And the dad's turned up.' She takes a long suck on her fag. 'Fifteen years old, barely capable of tying his own shoelaces.'

'Right.'

'And he's asking for a paternity test.'

'What? I'm amazed he knows the word.'

'I get the feeling he's seen it on *Jeremy Kyle* or *Trisha* or something like that, and he didn't actually use the word, he just said he knew his rights and he wanted a test.'

'So, all sweetness and light in Maternity this afternoon!'

'No more than usual,' she smiles. 'Anyway, I'm off out this afternoon. Doing my rounds.'

'That should be nice,' I say, looking up at a relatively blue sky. 'A bit of fresh air.'

'You say that,' she says, 'but I can't say I enjoy trawling through all those estates knocking on doors. Don't get me wrong, the people are nice enough, it's just that all those flats are so small and shitty. Actually, they're not really flats. They're rooms that they've sub-let off some council tenant. So what should be a council house with two bedrooms now has something like five different families, one to a room, making about twenty people all living in a two-bed flat and some tosspot somewhere earning five hundred a month per family. It's amazing. They've a bed but nothing to really sit on, maybe a sofa, but always, without fail, they have a plasma TV. I don't know how or where they get one, but they've all got one. Nothing to eat, but they've got a plasma. Nowhere to sit, but they've got a plasma. It's like the other thing I always see. Really expensive buggies – Bugaboos, that sort of thing.'

'I'm not sure I know what they look like,' I say.

'Oh you know, Gwyneth Paltrow had one and now they're what all the mums want. That's what they spend their five-hundred-quid Surestart maternity grant on.'

'What grant?'

'After a certain stage in your pregnancy you get assessed and then you get given it, along with the hundred-and-ninety-quid Health and Pregnancy grant that everyone gets.'

'What? And they spend all that money at once on a pushchair?'

'Most of it,' she says, taking a final drag before dropping the butt on the ground and crushing it with her foot. 'Well, at least they're spending it on the baby.'

'God,' I say, feeling depressed.

'I have got very used to going into smelly crowded houses. There are always a lot of children living in these cramped conditions, which of course doesn't help.'

'It all sounds very Victorian to me.'

'It is. Except for the Bugaboo and the plasma. The thing is, they have access to the healthcare system but no access to the welfare state. They're mostly illegal. They don't work, they can't work. I'm not really sure how they survive.'

'Aren't you scared going down there?'

'Most people are usually nice,' Mary replies. 'I am, after all, a woman who is coming round to look at their baby. But I have seen some really shocking things. People do love their babies, but their ability to look after them . . .' She shakes her head. 'Last week I saw a baby with a bottle taped to its mouth. It was a tiny newborn, with all this Sellotape around its mouth; it could barely move or breathe. I wasn't sure whether it was done out of laziness or just to shut it up. I did report that to Social Services. But, you know, it's hard. Some people don't have a clue.'

Mary goes on to tell me that some parents think they can start putting tea in the bottle after a couple of weeks. Give it some cow's milk, maybe with a bit of flour in it to fill it up. This is one of the reasons why the government has upped the weaning age from four to six months, because people feed their kids so badly; they thought that if they kept babies on milk a little longer they might get a better start. Not that it makes much difference, apparently. All that happens is those who were going to feed their kids KFC still do, and those who were going to give them organic carrots wait that bit longer. Although two months is the average age at which the KFC brigade wean their babies. No wonder, then, that we have an obesity problem.

'The people I deal with are so far removed from the people making the laws or coming up with these ideas and plans,' Mary continues. 'They think the rules don't apply to them. They live completely outside society.'

'And what are you doing this afternoon?'

'Weighing, heel-prick tests, that sort of thing. Testing for sickle-cell anaemia. You know, the usual.'

'I don't envy you at all,' I say, exhaling a plume of smoke into the sky.

'Yeah, well, everyone has to be checked, even the mums who are completely white and don't stand a chance of having sickle cell. You never know who the dad is.'

An estate car pulls up in front of us and a very large, very red-faced, puffing woman hauls herself slowly and gingerly out of the passenger seat. A rather more frantic-looking man/partner/husband has whipped out of the driving seat and is helping her. The woman leans against the car to catch her breath while the bloke scurries to the boot to pull out a suitcase, a bucket, another bag and a giant silver ball. Somehow he manages to carry or get hold of all these items and lock the car with his keys.

'OK, darling,' he says over the top of the silver ball, 'can you walk?'

'One minute.' She huffs and pants and puffs and exhales. She is clearly riding quite a big contraction. 'OK,' she squeaks. 'I think I can move now.'

'If she's not careful she'll be a born-before-arrival in the car park,' I say to Mary.

'Either that or she's about one centimetre dilated,' Mary responds, looking the woman up and down as she and her man/partner/husband list their way towards the front doors of the hospital. 'She's got the whole NCT thing going.'

National Childbirth Trust women are famous for arriving with their balls, buckets and birth plans that usually involve scented oils, smelly candles and a lot of moaning, groaning and tantric massage. In my experience, with all this comes a deep distrust or, at best, wariness of hospitals in general. So they are also prone to cleaning the birthing room from top to bottom as well as the lavatory, and some have been known to eschew the hospital's clear plastic cribs for a brought-from-home Moses basket. Having read every book on the subject of birth and having also got intimately in touch with themselves doing yoga, they can also be very dismissive of us lot. I remember one couple telling Julian off for checking the heart monitor, telling him to stop bothering them, like he was some desperate pregnancy perv gagging to be in the room with them or something.

These guys seem to have drawn the line at the Moses basket but they have all the other NCT paraphernalia, including what looks like an iPod for the inevitable pan pipes, whale noises or World Music collection.

'She'll be demanding an epidural in about half an hour,' says Mary. 'I'd better get out of here before I have to get PC Patsy over there a great big shot of pethidine.'

'I thought that was banned.'

'It is.'

'I always thought it was strange to tell women that they're not allowed to drink during pregnancy only to whack the baby with a whole load of opiates just as it comes into the world, leaving it too stoned to breastfeed. Although I could think of worse ways to arrive.'

'True.' She smiles. 'See you later.'

'Good luck,' I say. 'I may not see you before I go. I'm leaving today.'

'Of course.' She nods. 'Black Wednesday tomorrow.' She gives a little shiver. 'I'll see you around.' She gives me a wave and walks off.

Back in A&E, all the cubicles and most of the private rooms are full. The majority of the curtains are closed but I can see a young bloke dressed in tennis gear with some sort of twist or break to his ankle. Opposite him is a middle-aged woman in a floral frock sitting up reading *Hello!* She's flicking through the pages like she's waiting for a pedicure at a beauty salon. She is waiting, it transpires, after I ask Andrea, for a repeat prescription for HRT. Hardly an A&E problem, but apparently her doctor's on holiday and she's desperate.

Over at the far end there seems to be a bit of a queue for the computer. Jon Berry doesn't appear to want to move his skinny pre-pubescent arse from the area, and he's been joined by someone else.

'Who the hell is that?' I ask Ian, who is ambling past with a fist full of bloods.

'Oh Christ,' he says, rolling his small bloodshot eyes. 'It's another one of those tosspots.'

I continue to look quizzical. 'That doesn't narrow it down.'

'Oh you know, a tosspot, a management consultant – from Accenture or McKinsey or wherever.'

'What? Another person's been sent to scrabble around and try to find more bloody cuts and shavings?'

'It's like inviting vampires to the blood bank,' says Ian.

'It would help if they actually spoke to the staff,' I suggest.

'No one asks us *anything*!' says Ian. 'It's the NHS!'

Too true. No one ever asks our opinion on anything. Just a

thought, but perhaps they should have chatted to a few doctors before embarking on the multi-billion-pound overhaul of our computer system, instead of giving the go-ahead to the programme after what was a 'sofa meeting' without any consultation with doctors or any other members of staff about what might be useful, practical or indeed helpful in some way. Instead, the government blithely went ahead and embarked on the largest non-military IT project in the world, at a cost of £12.7 billion, only for it to fall flat on its face some eight years later, having cost us over £400 million. Think of the beds and drugs and man hours that figure equates to. But, you know, what's a few billion when you have a grand scheme to accomplish?

Then again, waste is the order of the day in a monolith like the NHS. It's the boring things that are annoying when you work here. Sterilized swabs only coming in packs of five, so you use two and have to throw the rest away. Scissors that are only used once before they too must be discarded, when they could be sterilized and reused. Drugs coming in the wrong packets and sizes. I am forever opening vials of lidnocaine, a local anaesthetic, using one-tenth of it, and throwing the rest away. But what are you supposed to do? The organization is so huge that the idea of catering to individuals is too expensive. It's like working in some old Soviet factory where it's easier to keep the gas burner burning all day rather than turn it on and off, because they have run out of matches. It's the same logic in the NHS. It's too difficult to sterilize a pair of scissors so let's just use them once then chuck them in the bin.

Talking of waste, I suddenly notice Mr Lee sitting bolt upright in Andrea's office. His briefcase is resting on the desk next to the chocolates, and he's staring expectantly at the door.

'What's happening with Mr Lee?' I ask Ian, before he wanders off.

'Oh, I know,' he replies. 'Poor sod, I think they're trying to find some sort of use for him. Andrea's on the case. They are after a position where he doesn't have to talk to patients or interact very much at all.'

'Pathology?' I suggest.

'Or the morgue. There are always openings in the morgue.'

'He could always earn a living translating for patients on the ward. D'you remember that other Chinese doctor we had who was discovered moonlighting as a translator on the wards?'

'I think that requires you to have at least a rudimentary grasp of English,' suggests Ian.

'Oh yeah.' My brain is very slow today. 'I'd better go and check up on a patient.'

'Your hip woman is still in the corridor,' he says as he walks off.

Shit! June! I presumed she'd been taken care of hours ago. Last I heard, Margaret was looking for an orthopod to check her hip and she'd been sent for an X-ray.

I open the corridor door to find her lying there, looking very stiff and grey. Her X-ray results are sitting on the end of her bed, but no one had told me they were back, or that the consultant had not arrived. I feel awful. Not as awful as her, obviously. But awful just the same.

'Hello, June,' I say, 'I am so sorry you've been left here. How are you?'

Her face slowly turns to look at me. She looks terrible, like she is in a lot of pain and has been for some time. I check her IV and her fluids bag is empty. Shit. What the hell is going on here? While the rest of us have been chasing our own arses next door, June has been lying here in agony and no one has noticed.

'I don't feel terribly well,' she says. Her eyes are looking a little cloudy. She is probably dehydrated and needs a strong painkiller right away. 'I think I would like to see a priest.'

'A priest? Really, June, I don't think it has come to that,' I say, trying to be jolly as I take hold of her wrist. It feels floppy, and her pulse is weak. I can feel my own pulse increasing rapidly. This is not just your usual dehydration. 'I'll just go and get a nurse.'

'Don't leave me,' she says, her voice sounding very feeble indeed.

'I'll be back in a minute, I promise.'

I march straight back into A&E, throwing back the doors. Andrea stands and stares at me like I'm some melodramatic thesp on the set of *ER*.

'All right, sunshine?' she says, somewhat disparagingly.

'No, I am not. I have a patient in her seventies who might be dying in the corridor.' I want to scream but I manage to control myself, so my words come out as some sort of quiet, spitting rage.

'What, out there?' Andrea says, seeing *Daily Mail* headlines flash up before her.

I have never seen such a short, large woman shift so quickly in my life. Before I can turn round to follow her she's through the door and by June's side, assessing the situation.

'All right, dear?' she says, tapping the back of June's hand. 'How are you?'

June is so weak that she can't be bothered to castigate Andrea for her slow, patronizing question, like she did with me when she first came in. The fight is going out of her. Where are her children? I pump back up the IV and hope that the drugs might make her feel a bit better.

'I would like to see a priest,' says June, quietly but clearly. 'As soon as possible, please.'

I look at Andrea and she looks at me. We both know that this is not looking good. Or at least June is not looking good. We have a prayer room in the hospital, which is multi-denominational, and we have a chaplain who visits the wards on a Thursday, I think it is. And he does sometimes give Holy Communion to those who want it. But we are at the heart of a big city and we all live much more secular lives. We don't have a priest on tap to talk to the sick or dying.

'I'm going to get Ian and Chris Williams,' I announce.

'And I'll stay right here,' says Andrea, squeezing June's ever more feeble hand.

It takes another ten minutes for June to die. She never did get her priest. What she got was Ian tap-dancing on her chest, trying to massage her heart back into action. She got armfuls of adrenalin, she got Chris shouting out orders left and right, and she got nurses struggling to get more lines into her narrow veins, jabbing away at her tissue-thin skin. It was not a quiet death and it was not dignified. It was a mad scramble to the end, with everyone trying their best to eke out another few days, weeks or even months for June. Most of all, no one wanted her to die here. On our watch. Of a heart attack. Andrea and Chris are worried about their statistics. We have on average about five deaths a week here. We're on target this week as June is the first death so far and it's already Tuesday.

You can't say that it doesn't affect you, because it does. When you first qualify you take every death personally and you can remember exactly how or why and what their names were, but obviously the more deaths you see, the less they affect you. You come to expect grannies to die at bus stops and old boys to slip over on the ice, but if they arrive talking and compos mentis through the doors and you strike up a conversation with them, like I did with June, then you are hit a little harder when they go.

I remember a mate who was asked about the point at which a hospital death became a tragedy saying, 'When they are younger than you.' So anyone coming in here who dies under the age of thirty is obviously going to affect me more than, say, some sixty-five-year-old with pneumonia. Then again, the circumstances of the death, or the way they speak or look, or an attitude they have, or just their age, can remind you of a friend, brother, father or lover, and then you are ten times more likely to be affected. Earlier this year an old boy came in who was the spitting image of my dad. He had a blocked bowel and died five days later of inoperable cancer. He was a little bit gruff, like my dad, and couldn't express himself very well, just like my dad, and when he died I found myself shedding a tear for him in the Gents. It was very weird.

Obviously children and babies are the worst. We had an eleven-year-old boy die back in March when I was still new here and I found it very hard to be on my own for a couple of days. I wanted to sort of offload some of my thoughts and

119

opinions but no one else was interested. There's always a departmental debrief after a child dies, so that everyone can have a say about what they are feeling, but no one ever does. They just head off home as early as they can and drink a bit more vodka than usual.

When babies die there is a whole protocol that staff have to follow. Upstairs they oversee between six and seven thousand births a year, and a couple of babies die each week. They hope not to get any dead mothers, but about three or four a year don't make it. After twenty-four weeks of gestation a stillbirth is viewed as a baby that requires a proper burial; before twenty-four weeks it is clinical waste and is more or less treated as such. After twenty-four weeks, the birth and the death have to be registered at the same time, and the chaplain is called. The baby is dressed and put in a room and the parents are encouraged to go and see it and take photographs so that they can begin to mourn it properly. Or so the current philosophy goes. Some women know their babies are going to die and give birth to them fully aware that they have only a few hours at the most, say because their child has an incurable heart condition. But for some it comes as a complete shock. There is still so much that is not picked up on the scans.

'Time of death?' says Chris as he starts to fill in June's paperwork.

'Fourteen fifty-eight,' I say.

'Does anyone know if she wants to be cremated?' asks Ewan, who has apparently appeared from nowhere.

'You greedy little sod,' says Ian, wiping the sweat off his forehead. 'I think I need some air.'

3–4 p.m.

Poor old Ewan. He was only asking the same question many of us hard-up student doctors have asked over the years. There was no need for Ian to make him feel so grubby about it.

'What?' says Ewan, two huge patches of red bursting across his cheeks. 'Someone's got to do it!'

And he's right. Someone does have to sign her death certificate, go through all her notes and release her to the undertakers. And whoever signs all the papers has to check that if she wants to be cremated she hasn't got a pacemaker. If they don't check properly and the crematorium blows up as a result they are liable for the first £10,000 worth of damage. For their pains they will get paid £71. Well, actually two doctors have to sign the certificate and they are paid £142. It's the dead person's family, or the deceased's estate, who pays. Normally it is part of the costs charged to the family by the undertaker.

'Ash cash', as it is rather pleasantly referred to, is one of the perks of being a junior doctor. It's a way of supplementing your income and ensuring a few more drunken nights out. Each hospital has its own system when it comes to ash cash. The last place I was at there was a very clear pecking order. If it was your patient who died then you were entitled to the money, and if you weren't in or were away on holiday then the person below you got to sign. You were supposed to give a tenner to the Mess Fund to help towards one of the numerous piss-ups, and the rest you could keep. Other hospitals pool the whole lot into the Mess Fund for everyone to enjoy. Here it's a bit more of a free-for-all, which can lead to the rather un-dignified sight of a scrum of junior doctors around a tepid corpse.

'You are very welcome to sign the certificate, if you want,' I say to Ewan. Quite frankly I have better things to do with my time, and I'm also slightly upset, to be honest, that June, who presented as such a robust patient, could go down so quickly. 'Remember, you'll only get the cash if she's cremated in the end, and only after about two or three months. So don't go spending it all at once.'

'Well, actually, I was thinking I might put it towards a holiday,' says Ewan.

'A holiday! On June!' says Ian. 'I'm sure she'd be delighted to know that her passing helped you to bang three Es and large it with your mates on a podium in Ibiza.'

'I wasn't planning on going to Ibiza,' Ewan counters.

'Really,' says Ian, clicking the top of his pen in and out in irritation. 'Where's June sending you then?'

'Australia.'

'I'm sure she'd be delighted to know that—'

'I saved up for a computer with my ash cash,' Louise chips in.

'A computer!' I exclaim, staring at her.

'Yup,' she nods. 'It took ten deaths but I got it in the end.'

'Only ten!' declares Ian, his small red eyes now totally spherical.

'Well,' says Louise, 'I didn't want to drink it so I thought I would do something useful with it. I needed a computer to pass my exams so I thought that would be a good thing to spend it on. I thought they would approve. I do remember most of the people who died when I use it.'

'What?' says Ian. 'You think of Maureen while you chat to your mates on Facebook?'

'I'm not on Facebook,' Louise responds.

'Aren't you?' asks Ewan.

'There has to be at least one perk for working in Oncology,' she says. 'Anyway, what did you spend your ash cash on, then, Ian? Booze and fags?'

'Booze and fags,' he confirms.

'And that's *so* much more fitting, don't you think?' she purrs before walking back into the department.

'She needs a good shag, that girl,' says Ian.

I am just about to offer my services to the lovely Louise when Andrea pokes her head through the doors and says, 'There's a Mrs Maynard to see you.'

My heart sinks. Poor Mrs Maynard. The very sad Mrs Maynard. I do feel sorry for the woman but she is driving me

crazy with her mad obsession. About a month ago Mrs
Maynard lost her son, Paul. He was obviously once a nice
young man who loved his mum and remembered her birthday,
but sadly he became a desperate, grubby, rank old crackhead
who sold his life and soul for rocks and who eventually died of
a crack-induced heart attack in a crack den about ten streets
away from here. Anyway, between the crack den and A&E the
paramedics performed mouth-to-mouth and CPR and in all the
trauma and the battle Paul lost his T-shirt. And Mrs Maynard
wants it back. This is the fourth time she has come asking for
it and I am afraid that my sympathy wanes a little more each
time I see her. I understand that she is miserable at the loss of
her son. That she is upset and wants something to remind her
of him. But a stinking, filthy crack-shirt covered in spittle and
vomit is not the answer. Nor, indeed, do we have it. I have
looked high and low for the foul and fetid thing, to no avail.
She has written to the hospital, I have had meetings about the
T-shirt, but there is no way I can magically find something that
has been lost for a month now. She has even apparently been
staking out the crack house, trying to get in and search it in the
hope of finding her son's top. It is sad, desperate, and bloody
annoying.

I take a deep breath.

'Good afternoon, Mrs Maynard,' I say, trying to be charming and positive.

The poor woman looks frantic and distraught. Her thin
brown hair hangs lank and unwashed from a centre parting
and her clothes look like they haven't seen any Persil for weeks.
Her gaunt face looks grey and there are large red bags under

her eyes. If I didn't know she was a staunch Seventh-Day Adventist I would swear she was on the crack herself.

'Is it good?' she asks, her hands and fingers tying themselves in knots.

'Well, perhaps not,' I say.

'I have left you messages,' she starts.

'Oh really? I'm very sorry, I haven't got them.'

Weirdly, I'm not lying. The message system in this place is shit. I have more or less accepted that I am completely un-contactable at work; it's like living and working in some sort of bubble. The real world goes on outside and occasionally crashes in, mostly on a stretcher, but I do my shift and then emerge blinking into the light at the end of it, like a small myopic mole.

'Well, I've left you more than six,' she says, counting them off on her fingers.

'I am sorry,' I say, taking a step towards her. She recoils, like I'm about to do her serious harm. 'Would you like a cup of tea?'

'A cup of tea?'

Oh no, I think, what have I said now?

'My son is dead and all you offer me is a cup of tea?' Some colour is coming back to her cheeks.

'No, no, I was just wondering if you want a cup of tea while we talked about your son,' I try. I'm really not very good at this.

'I don't want a cup of tea,' she shrieks, 'I want my son's T-shirt, which you have stolen!'

'I haven't stolen your son's T-shirt, Mrs Maynard.' I'm

125

trying to be consolatory. I'm not sure it's working. 'It was lost on the way here in the ambulance.'

'I have been in contact with the police,' she continues, her head wobbling with defiance, 'and I am going to have you charged with theft.' She jabs the air with a skinny white finger. 'Theft! Do you hear? Theft!'

'OK, that's fine,' I say, ushering her towards the exit. 'I'll be very happy to talk to the police when they get here.'

'They won't be coming to talk to you, they'll be coming to arrest you!'

'OK then, arrest me. I'll look forward to that.'

'So will I!' she yells as she marches off. 'You're a thief, doctor! You are nothing more than a thief who steals from dead people!'

She walks out of the building, leaving me standing in the waiting room with about thirty pairs of eyes staring at me. Some of them are looking at me in befuddled amusement; others clearly believe her story and are staring at me with indignation. All I can do is smile and shrug my shoulders. Anything I say will only sound hollow.

I walk back into A&E and send a bloke with a suspected broken toe up to X-ray and dress a cooking burn before I am approached by a smirking Steve. He's standing there grinning at me, his blue eyes shining, as he runs his hands through his thick dark hair.

'Woman,' he says, with a sniff. 'Cubicle three – I need a second opinion.'

'Really?' I say. I'm feeling tetchy and quite frankly have better things to do.

'Yup,' he smiles. 'Just check the apex pulse, please.'

'Apex?'

'Apex.' He smiles and taps the side of his nose. So I poke my head around the curtain and smile. 'Excuse me, Mrs . . . ?'

A well-preserved woman of about sixty raises her head off the pillow. 'Ms Evans,' she says.

'Excuse me, Ms Evans. Would you mind if I repeated the pulse check my colleague here has just carried out? He's asking me for a second opinion.'

'No, go ahead,' she says, unbuttoning her shirt to reveal a very striking, somewhat unexpectedly ample bosom and a shocking pink and purple lace push-up bra.

'I'm very sorry about this,' I say, rounding my hand and cupping her firm, full bosom. I squeeze it and feel around underneath for a pulse, checking its rate, rhythm and strength. 'Well, that all seems fine to me.' I nod to her to button up her cream cotton top. 'Thank you very much.'

'No problem, doctor,' she says.

I close the curtain behind me only to turn round slap-bang into Steve, who is now grinning broadly.

'Well?' he whispers. 'What do you think?'

'The pulse seems fine to me.'

'Not the pulse, you idiot, the tits!'

'What do you mean, "the tits"?'

'Aren't they cracking?' He nods and grins like an oversexed schoolboy. 'Quite spectacular!'

'Jesus Christ, Steve, what the hell is wrong with you? She's a hundred and five!'

'Actually she's sixty-three. It must be one of the earliest boob jobs on record.'

They were amazing, I have to agree. They must have been very expensive in their day. Not the usual knobbly-knees cheap tits we often see around here.

'Whoever did them did a good job,' I admit finally.

'You've got to love a TUBE,' says Steve.

'A TUBE?'

'Yup.' He nods.

'What the hell was she in for?'

'Twisted her knee!' He laughs. 'She didn't seem to mind!'

A TUBE, or totally unnecessary breast examination, is one of Steve's favourite shticks. He fancies himself as a bit of a breast connoisseur, having felt up half the country. Well, him and half the junior doctors on staff. If they think they can get away with a TUBE, they will slip one in, so to speak, and no one ever really notices or even thinks to complain. Steve maintains that it is one of the perks of the job. It jollies up his day. He puts on his best doctor face, speaks in his VTMK (voice to melt knickers – a voice deliberately cultivated by some doctors), and no one is any the wiser. He likes doing that sort of thing, taking the piss slightly. He's also one for laughing or having a good look at a body when it's out cold on the slab. He is liable to drag a colleague out of a consultation just to have a cop at someone's interesting pubic hair, a ridiculously small or large penis, or a huge pair of breasts. He's also very fond of a piercing, which are two a penny in Gynaecology. The number of times you have to ask women in labour to take out clitoral piercings is extraordinary. I imagine he will find himself a little bereft of entertainment when he goes up north to do paediatrics. It won't be nearly so diverting.

Although doctors can usually find some means of entertaining themselves. If you look carefully on your notes, you will see they are littered with acronyms, or little jokes between staff. There are the old ones, like NFN (Normal for Norfolk) and FLK (Funny-Looking Kid), for those patients whose looks and behaviour are a little strange. Odd- or ugly-looking babies often have ILWF on the bottom of their charts, which means In Line With Family. There are others, like E17 or Barking, which means the patient is obviously bonkers, and TTFO (Told to Fuck Off), which means the patient is difficult. TSL – Too Stupid to Live. TFTB – Too Fat to Breathe. There are other codes in referral letters that serve as warnings. For instance, a doctor referring to a patient as 'interesting' or 'complex' in a case letter is telling the other doctor to run a mile. My personal favourite, which I have only seen twice in my career so far, is TFBUNDY – Totally Fucked But Unfortunately Not Dead Yet.

I leave Steve to enjoy his little joke a bit longer and head off to the computer to get my next presentation. David the clean-shaven keen-faced general plastic surgeon is back from checking out the burns victim and is talking to Chris.

'So what have you got on your list this afternoon?' asks Chris, leafing through some X-rays.

'More skin cancer,' replies David, rolling his little brown eyes. 'It's just so not challenging. I can do it with my eyes shut.'

'You can't do the big stuff all the time,' says Chris, holding a sheet up to the ceiling strip light.

'I know, I know,' David says, cracking his fingers. 'But it

doesn't stop you wishing. Last week I had a twenty-two-hour operation, a woman with a tumour so large it was like an alien coming out of her stomach. She said she'd only had it for a couple of weeks, but they all say that, don't they? A couple of weeks, when what they really mean is five years. Because this thing had actually burst through the stomach lining and the skin and was sticking out like a stalagmite, and that simply can't have taken two weeks!'

'Twenty-two hours?' says Chris, looking impressed.

'You have a bacon sandwich to get yourself going and then, you know, you pop out when you want, just so long as there's an anaesthetist. They're warm and asleep, what does it matter?'

'You could pop home and watch *EastEnders*!' jokes Jon Berry, butting in.

'No,' says David, looking at him like he's an idiot. Then he picks up where he left off. 'It's not so much the tumour that takes all the time, it's the hole we have to fill afterwards.'

'I can imagine,' says Chris, who I can tell has already lost interest.

'Me? I'm a fan of the thigh when it comes to filling holes. You can get all you want from the thigh. Skin, flesh, muscle, fat, blood supply – it's all there. Just slice it off and attach all the veins. Brilliant. There's a surgeon I know, James Kerr. Do you know him?'

'Hummm . . .' Chris is pretending to search through his memory banks.

'Well, he's amazing, he can fill any hole in the history of holes. There isn't a hole he can't fill.'

'Your cakehole?' Steve mutters as he walks past.

'What?' asks David, turning round and looking bemused.

Poor old David, he's just like all the other plastic surgeons I know: obsessive and overachieving. It's almost like they have an extra six hours in the day over the rest of us. I know one bloke who drives a very nice Maserati who decided four years ago that he wanted to take up diving, and then three years ago he took up underwater photography. Last month he had two seahorse photos in *National Geographic*. No one was in the least bit surprised. They are all geniuses who verge on the insane. This same surgeon will only operate to Elvis, and will always close, in so much as he does his own stitching, to 'Return to Sender' (he once had an operation that was going badly until that track came on, and now he always uses it). Rumour also has it that he used to put his cigar through the Central Sterile Supply Department so that he could chew on it during operations.

'Have you heard the joke about the two plastic surgeons talking to each other?' asks Chris.

'Sorry? No,' says David, looking even more confused than ever.

'One says to the other, "I had a vision just now that God came and spoke to me and said that I was the best surgeon who ever lived." And the other surgeon replied, "But I haven't spoken to you today."'

Chris laughs, even Jon Berry joins in with a little snigger, but David just stands there.

'Anyway,' he says, 'I'll just go and do the paperwork, but he looks OK for some grafts tomorrow, which should, you know, help with the hands. It'll take some time because it looks as if the petrol ran down his arm before anything else, but we can start, get cracking . . .'

'Good, good,' says Chris. 'You can use Andrea's office if you like. Ignore Mr Lee sitting in there. We're trying to find him a position in the hospital. You don't speak any Chinese, do you?'

'Me? No. A little Swahili, which I picked up when I was working in Africa. Amazing experience. I got four years' training in three months.' No one is listening to him now. 'In here, then?' he says slowly, wandering into Andrea's office.

I turn round to see Andrea coming towards me.

'Woman, cubicle two,' she says. 'She's a little pissed off.'

'They're always pissed off,' I say, searching for my user-friendly smile and gentle bedside manner.

Just over two hours left and counting.

'Good afternoon,' I say as breezily as I can when I get to the cubicle. I look down at the notes. 'Mrs Parker? What seems to be the problem?'

'The problem, mister,' says the obese woman sitting opposite me who has poured herself into a pair of black leggings and a large white T-shirt with a pink glitter Playboy bunny logo stretched across her huge bosom, 'is that we've been here for three hours.'

'Well, I'm very sorry about that,' I say. 'We have had a lot of poorly people in today. You're entitled to complain if it's over four hours.'

'Yeah, well, anyway, the thing is, Brandon here has got ADHD and we need the drugs for it.'

A neon-pink finger is pointing at an overweight boy in a pair of blue tracksuit bottoms who is sitting on a red plastic chair, his thighs seeping over the edge of the seat.

'ADHD?' I say, looking at Brandon, who looks as active as an atrophied blancmange. 'And what sort of symptoms is he having?'

'Umm,' says Mrs Parker, clearly trying to remember something. 'He has attention problems.'

'Ri-i-ight. And?'

'He is hyperactive. He has problems at school. His learning and that.'

'OK . . .'

I'm taking notes but I don't believe a word of it. Brandon couldn't look less hyperactive if he tried. His arms are folded across his soft stomach and he has a pair of breasts large enough to pique Steve's interest. Not that children with ADHD are necessarily slim, but they do tend not to be able to sit still, buttocks glued to a chair, particularly if they have been kept waiting for three hours.

'How old is Brendon?'

'Brandon.'

'Yes. How old is he?'

'Seven,' she says. 'And as sole carer I find it very hard to take care of him. I'm a single parent, you see. All three of my other children have ADHD . . .'

Mrs Parker continues with her story, which I am afraid I have heard a thousand times before. She knows what things to say to me, what boxes to tick for me to believe her. Except I don't. I had a heroin addict in last week trying the same scam, trying to convince me that her poor fifteen-year-old son had ADHD as well. Claim your child has ADHD and you are entitled to more benefits; play the system correctly and you siphon off an extra £10,000 a year. You claim through the Disability Living Allowance, which then entitles you to extra income support and extra child tax credits, and if you are really good you can get a carer's allowance thrown in as well. This goes some way towards explaining why only two thousand children were diagnosed with ADHD in 1991 but now some 5 per cent of children in the country suffer from the disorder, with one in five children in the state sector said to have 'special needs'. So while the parents pocket the cash to cater for their needs, their children end up taking drugs, like Ritalin, that they don't actually need.

I look at Brandon and his mum. They are examples of just one of the numerous social health issues that come into A&E on a daily basis. What Brandon needs is a better diet – some fruit and vegetables instead of endless sugars and carbo-hydrates – and some regular exercise. He is already obese at the age of seven; he'll probably be morbidly obese by the age of fifteen and he'll probably develop diabetes and other com-plications, dying of one of them in his late fifties. Coming from this arse end of town, his life expectancy is seventeen years lower than the richest members of our society. But it's not my place to advise someone like Mrs Parker on how to live her life and bring up her children.

If I give her a prescription for Brandon then I'm not being true to my training, or indeed my beliefs; if I don't, her life and Brandon's life remain difficult. So what do I do? I do what every good doctor does when faced with a tricky dilemma: I pass the buck.

'Mrs Parker,' I say, 'I would love to be able to help you and Brandon out, but I'm afraid this is a GP issue. We are Accident and Emergency, and Brandon, I'm afraid, is neither.'

'But,' she says, heaving herself out of her seat, 'I brought Kelly in here a few months back—'

'It's the system,' I say. 'What can I do?'

She looks at me, and as a connoisseur of the system, she immediately understands. She has played me and lost. She needs to try a little harder next time.

'I'll get my GP to sign the form then,' she says. 'He won't mind a bit.'

4–5 p.m.

As I escort Mrs Parker and Brandon through the door of the waiting room to scam another day, I bump into a rather attractive woman in her late forties just coming in. She is carrying a large box of expensive-looking chocolates and a bunch of pink peonies. She looks up and down the waiting room, which has emptied a bit since I was last here. The OAPs near the television appear to have wended their way home to catch *Countdown* in the comfort of their own sitting rooms, to be replaced by the usual sort of playground cuts and scrapes that are currently Ewan's (being the most junior) bread and butter.

The woman stands in the middle of the waiting room looking around. She clearly has no idea where she is supposed to be.

'Can I help you?' I ask.

'Um, I'm not sure,' she says. She is wearing a floral summer wrap dress that stops just below her knee, and blue flip-flops. Her blonde hair is tied in a ponytail. 'My mother was admitted here this morning. She's broken her hip. June Bartley? Old woman? Quite chatty?'

'June Bartley,' I say, trying to buy myself some time. 'And you are?' Though I already know the answer.

'Her daughter,' she replies.

'Right . . . um . . .'

'Audrey,' she says.

'Audrey,' I repeat. 'If you would like to follow me.'

'Oh, good.' She smiles. 'You know where she is, that's lucky. My neighbour told me I might be wandering around for hours. These places are so big, aren't they? Hospitals? Enormous! Well, I suppose they have to be, the amount of sick people we have.' She laughs. She is gabbling and clearly nervous. 'She's OK, though, isn't she? Mum? She's never had a fall before. So weird. She lives on her own, you see. Since Dad died. She doesn't want to live with us. Or the others. She much prefers it on her own. She's got her friends. She is all right, isn't she? Because her neighbour was a little bit doubtful. I said she's as strong as an ox. Mum. Strong as an ox.'

'If you'd like to wait in here,' I say, pointing to one of the empty rooms that we have with a door. 'I'll go and get someone to talk to you.'

I suppose I could have told her there and then that her mother was dead, but we've been taught to make sure people are sitting down and out of the way, just in case something kicks off. Also, I just don't feel in the mood to break her heart. I have less than two hours left and I just don't think I can cope with the questions, because I'm going to find it hard to answer them without telling her that her mother was lying on her own in a corridor for several hours and that she was my patient. I would much prefer Chris to tell her. People accept sad news much better from people with grey hair; they look distinguished and trustworthy. She doesn't want to hear about her mother's passing from someone who's got another half-century left.

Chris takes it in his stride when I ask him. After eight years in A&E he has become rather good at delivering bad news. I see him walk over to the consulting room and close the door.

'You OK?' asks Louise, surprising me from behind. 'Was that your NOF's daughter?'

'What?' I say, jumping slightly.

'Your hip fracture? Was that her daughter?'

'Yes. I think she is going to be very sad.'

'Do you want a cup of coffee?'

That is the first time in six months she has offered to get me anything. And I'm a little stunned. 'That's very kind of you.'

'Well, you know, last day and everything.'

I follow her to the common room.

'You excited about moving on?' she asks me.

'I can't wait not to be doing A&E. Where are you going?' Like I don't already know.

'St Thomas's.' She smiles, slightly apologetically, knowing that it's one of the top postings in the country. 'General surgery, and then I think, you know, I might go on to do max fax or plastics.'

'I'm sure you will,' I smile. 'You'll get the good references.'

'What's that supposed to mean?' she asks, reaching the kettle and flicking it on.

'Nothing. You know, just that you're good.'

'Good at what?' she says, raising her eyebrows.

'Being a doctor,' I say.

'Someone's a bit defensive,' says Steve, coming in behind.

The terrible thing about this common room is that there are two swing doors into it, which means that no conversation is ever private.

'I'm not defensive,' she says.

'Well, you should be.' He grins.

Why does he have to come in right now, just as Louise and I are about to have a proper chat? I'm sure I could have managed to secure her telephone number. He is so annoying. I have only got just under two hours left and he is raining on my bloody parade. Not that there was much of a parade going on. But there could have been, if he'd given me five minutes. I can be quite charming when I put my mind to it.

'Well, I'm not defensive,' she says, defensively.

Steve opens the fridge. 'There's never any chocolate when you need it.'

'Did you nick my KitKat?' she asks.

'No, I didn't nick your bloody KitKat,' Steve replies. 'Honestly, have you got your period?'

'What?' she says, watching him amble out of the common room. 'That man is a total prick!'

'I heard that!' he shouts back through the swinging door.

'Good!' she says, marching out of the room.

'She fancies him,' announces Andrea, who is sitting in the corner, her mouth full of Jaffa Cakes.

'I think he likes Margaret,' I say.

'Don't be silly,' she chortles. Bits of cake fly out of her mouth. 'Margaret is just one of those very giving girls.' She looks at me to see if I am understanding her. 'She has been generous to a few patients in the past, you know.'

'Really?' I frown. Is she saying what I think she is saying?

'Oh yes. Very generous and giving indeed.' She mouths the word 'fellatio' at me and taps the side of her nose, giving me another little nod.

I leave the common room a little confused. It seems to be all kicking off on my last day. So Louise fancies Steve but may or may not be doing the senior consultant. And if she is, is it just to further her career? She is an ambitious piece of work. On the other hand Margaret is blowing Steve, who possibly fancies Louise, but she blows everyone – Margaret, that is, not Louise.

When I get back to A&E, Ewan, who is looking a little pale, grabs me.

'Mate,' he swallows. 'There's a DSH in resus one. Can you take it? I just can't cope with that amount of blood.'

A deliberate self-harm, or suicide attempt, presentation does tend to get a doctor's back up. There's enough shit going on without someone giving us extra work on purpose. It does tend to annoy us and make us a little unsympathetic. Particularly as there are so many repeat offenders. We have one woman who comes in here practically every other day having taken twenty paracetamol. Not enough to kill her, just enough to make her really rather poorly. It would bugger her liver if we did nothing, so we have to go through the motions, pumping her stomach and flushing her blood until it has all disappeared, only for her to come back a few days later having done the same thing all over again. You can imagine how popular she is round here. Even the resident psych team are bored witless by her.

But then she is, of course, only really seeking attention, crying for help. Men are much more successful than women when it comes to killing themselves. Although we get broadly the same number of attempts in through our doors, the male suicide rate of 17.7 per 100,000 is over triple that of women, which is only 5.4 per 100,000. Weirdly, it was the over-seventy-fives who used to account for most suicides in blokes, money problems and loneliness being the most obvious reasons, but that has changed recently: young men between fifteen and forty-four are now much more likely to kill themselves – for, I imagine, the same reasons. Women are more likely to kill themselves in middle age, between forty-five and seventy-four.

This patient appears to be a young woman in her early twenties.

'Her name is Katie Heywood,' says Connie, one of the more outgoing of the Filipina nurses. She reels off her BP, temperature and stats (blood oxygen saturation).

'Hello, Katie, can you hear me?' I begin.

She moves her head slightly. A curl of mouse-brown hair falls across her white, spotty face.

'Can you hear me, Katie? You're in hospital. You are still alive.'

I pick up her left arm, which has been bound tightly by the ambulance crew. Judging by the number of scars and lines all the way up her arm, she appears to be a dab hand at this self-harming lark. She has at least twenty scarred cut marks on this arm alone. I pick up the right arm and it's a similar story. Looking at all of this, I'm not sure if in this case she was meaning to kill herself or was just cutting herself again. But I have a feeling the latter is more likely. I snip away at the bandages that have been expertly tied by the ambulance crew and check the wound. It is deep and long and very bloody, but by the look of things she hasn't had the required strength actually to cut completely through the artery. Like most people who attempt to slash their wrists she has only nicked the main vein rather than spliced the whole thing open.

I have to say I have learnt to be wary of young females who attempt suicide. During one of my first rotations I was placed on Psychiatry in a rather small provincial hospital where I was a non-resident on call for twenty-four hours at a time. A young woman came in who had attempted to slash her wrists and I was asked to stitch her up. Then about an hour later I got another call saying that she had done it again and could I come and re-stitch her. The psychiatric nurses had their hands tied really. They were not allowed to do very much, all they could do was stand by and watch her cut herself again. While I was talking to the nurses about what to do if she attempted to cut herself again, we got a call saying that she had tried to hang herself. She was put into solitary, but the next day she tried to hang herself again using a sheet that she had wrapped around her neck and pulled with her foot like a tourniquet. However,

142

as she pulled with the foot, the sheet tightened and she passed out, and the foot lost its strength. It is, in fact, impossible to kill yourself using this method. But we took away her sheets anyway. By day three this was developing into a serious and deadly game of cat and mouse. She was developing a fixation on me and was using ever more elaborate ways to get my attention. She started to goad me, telling me that I was rubbish and didn't know my job. I was newly qualified so perhaps she had a point. The whole thing eventually became untenable when she stashed a sharp in the loo, and having persuaded a nurse that she could be trusted on her own, she locked the door and started shouting for me, telling me how shit I was, that she was going to do it again. She was trying to draw me into her vortex, drag me into her game. I have to say it was one of the hardest few days of my career. In the end she didn't manage to kill herself. She was sectioned and became somebody else's problem.

Connie tells me that she has already called the rapid response psych team to come down and evaluate Katie to see if she needs to be kept in under the Mental Health Act on a section 5.2 (for short-term assessment). Although these guys don't have the best track record, and I have had a few run-ins with them in the past. A few months ago I had a drunk tramp come in with a suspected overdose. This bloke was a bit of an A&E regular; the police had found him a few times in the past slumped in a doorway, and had brought him in to sober up. But this time he had taken an overdose, paracetamol as well as alcohol; it was not his normal behaviour. He had also been found on a train track waiting to be hit by a passing train. So I called the psych team to try to keep him in and assess him for twenty-four hours, as the man clearly needed help. The team came, checked him over, and said that he was perfectly OK to go home. I told them he lived on the streets. They said that he was fine to go back out on to the streets. They promised me that they would check up on him in a week, that they would find out where he was and bring him in for assessment. I warned them that he might attempt suicide again but they insisted he was fine. So he was released, there was nothing I could do to stop it. Two hours later he was found dead on the tracks. He'd walked straight out of A&E and straight under a train. I was livid, and of course I felt awful. I'd tried to do something but no one was listening. That sort of thing happens a lot around here.

But you know, sometimes we manage to turn things around. Sometimes even the most determined suicide attempt can be thwarted. I remember Louise telling me about a bloke who swallowed two litres of vodka, knocked back umpteen paracetamol and Prozac, and slit his wrists before getting into a car to drive to Beachy Head. He clearly meant to kill himself. Unfortunately (or fortunately) for him, he bled so much that his blood pressure dropped and he passed out at the wheel. He came to A&E as an RTA (road traffic accident) rather than an attempted suicide and was completely furious when we revived him. He'd had a row with his wife and wanted to finish it. Amazingly, the wife came to his bedside and they made up. They left together a few days later. He was apparently very grateful for this second chance.

I wonder how pleased Katie will be when she comes completely to.

A very slim, mousy-looking woman pokes her head around the curtains. 'Is she OK? I'm her mother.'

'She's fine,' I smile, covering up the wound with a swab. 'She's lost a bit of blood, but—'

'I do wish she would stop doing this,' Katie's mother says, mincing her thin pale hands. 'I blame her boyfriend. She hasn't been the same since she hooked up with him. She was good at school, you know, and was going to university until he came along, and now look.'

'Mum? Mum?' Katie moans, and rolls about on the bed. 'Go away, Mum. Why don't you go away?'

'It's your own fault all this!' the mother snaps. 'Told you that Danny wasn't good enough for you!'

'Go away, Mum.'

'No, I won't! Not until I have had my say!'

'Mum! Go away!'

'Um, perhaps it's better if you wait through there,' I say.

'Are you trying to get rid of me?' She looks at me, her top lip slightly curled to reveal a set of yellow rat teeth.

'I just think it would be better if you waited through there while I stitch up Katie and you can perhaps calm down a bit and then come back when she might be more ready for visitors.'

'I am not a visitor! I am her mother!'

'I know, I know,' I say, staring at Connie, urging her to do something.

'Would you like a cup of tea?' asks Connie, walking forward and putting her arm around the mother.

'A cup of tea?' She looks a little suspicious.

'Yes. With milk and sugar.'

Connie escorts the woman out of the cubicle and the tension dissipates.

Katie doesn't say a word while I stitch her up. She doesn't offer any explanation, and I don't bother to ask. I have had quite a day and am really looking forward to putting my feet up this evening and perhaps having some dinner with my girl-friend Emma. I'm hungry. Pizza would be nice. I put the finishing touches to Katie's bandage. She doesn't smile or say thank you. She simply rolls over and faces the wall. I hope the psych team get more out of her when they turn up.

Outside in the corridor there has been a change of shift for the SO19 officers. We have two new blokes wandering around A&E, cluttering up the area. I think two of our gangsters have been transferred to private rooms upstairs, which seems an ironic reward for bad behaviour. We only have one bloke left down here, awaiting transfer.

Chris is walking towards me; his face is a little drawn. I glance across at the door to the private room where June's daughter was sitting. It's open. A large box of chocolates and a bunch of pink peonies lie abandoned on a chair.

'How did she take it?' I ask, still staring at the flowers.

'Not well,' says Chris. 'She says she wants an inquiry, but I don't think she means it.'

'Really?'

I feel my heart racing a little, even though I know I did nothing wrong. Her mother may have lain in a corridor for a little too long, and she may have run out of fluids, but it wasn't actually my fault that she died. Heart failure due to the combination of stress from the fracture and the drugs is just one of those things. It's not something that we can predict or prevent. Then again, had I done something like given her too much morphine and plunged her into respiratory arrest, or given her too many fluids causing a heart attack, the results would have been similar. We look after our own in this hospital, so small mistakes, no matter how catastrophic, tend to . . . well, not exactly get brushed under the carpet, just not be highlighted exactly. If the mistakes are huge and catastrophic, the NHS will look after you. They won't fight your battle for you, they won't help you clear your name if it wasn't your fault, but they will always cough up for you and they will always settle out of court. Given the prospect of a protracted and expensive court case, the NHS would rather give the plaintiff half a million quid and tell them where to go. Which is obviously great if you are a shit doctor who is actually negligent, but if you are a good doctor who is being hounded or pursued by a vindictive nutter and his family it is less good, as you never get your day in court and have to carry on with your career slightly tarnished.

Of course there are some things, like a nurse killing several patients with an overdose of painkillers, that just can't be brushed aside; and neither can things like the persistent neglect of a patient that caused him to die after he had to telephone the hospital's switchboard begging for a glass of water, having been refused by a nurse. Then again some extraordinary stories, like a hospital porter having sex with patients as they were out cold on the trolley in the lift on their way to and from theatre, never see the light of day. This scandal was only unearthed after one of the patients became pregnant. Who knows how much the trust paid out then? Or how much it cost to put CCTV into all those lifts?

'I'm sure she doesn't mean it,' Chris says, giving my arm a squeeze. 'She's just upset. In my experience, she will go home and talk it over and realize that there was nothing to be done.'

'I hate it when that happens,' I say.

'I know.' He nods. 'So does that nice Mr Berry over there. Oh, by the way, have you seen our friend Mr Lee?'

'No.'

'That's annoying. We've managed to find him something in Pathology but we just can't seem to find him. His briefcase is still in the office.'

'He can't have gone far.'

'Let's hope not. Anyway, don't worry,' he says to me again, giving my shoulder a final squeeze before turning away.

I am just summoning the energy to go and see another patient – I'm sure I can fit in a couple more before I leave tonight – when Steve walks over.

'You look like you could do with cheering up,' he says. 'Follow me.'

I don't know why, but I follow him. It is true I could do with a laugh. He leads me through the double doors, along the corridor and off into the pre-med section just before theatre. Behind a curtain, lying on a trolley, anaesthetized to the world, is a young woman with dark brown hair. Beside her is Andy, sorting out his big syringe/little syringe combination.

'Not you again!' he says to Steve. 'Sod off!'

'You shouldn't have showed me if you didn't want me to share the joy,' says Steve.

'What?' I say.

'Take a look at this,' he says.

He lifts the bottom half of the woman's gown to reveal a Snoopy tattoo just above the bikini line. The character is grinning, pushing a lawn mower, cutting her pubic hair 'grass'.

'Isn't that magnificent?'

5–6 p.m.

Steve is going to get himself in real trouble one day. Undoubtedly Snoopy is very amusing, and if you are the sort of girl who puts a Snoopy tattoo just above your bush for comic effect then I'm pretty sure your intention is to have said tattoo admired and commented upon. However, I am also pretty sure that having your fanny sniggered at by five complete strangers while you are comatose and waiting to have your appendix cut out is not the kind of audience she'd envisaged. But I have only got an hour left in this place and I like Steve so I don't really want to part on bad terms. He's a good-looking bloke who will probably go far. I might need his help one day.

Back in A&E, poor Mr Lee has finally been located wandering around the ground floor. We think he went to find the loo and got lost trying to find his way back to the department, although no one is quite sure. Anyway, Chris very charmingly takes him under his wing and escorts him over to the lift, leaving Andrea to take him up to Pathology on the fifth floor.

'I wonder if we will ever see or hear of him again,' he says, standing by the computer, waiting for Jon Berry to finish whatever he's doing. 'Excuse me,' he says, scratching his greying hair in irritation, 'how much longer are you going to be?'

'I am just collating the waiting times for each patient today,' says Jon. His little pinhead appears to wobble with self-importance. 'And then we will combine the average with the other averages that have been gleaned over the past month and we can come up with a monthly average.'

'Right,' says Chris, inhaling with boredom. 'And meanwhile, what are we, the people actually looking after patients, supposed to do?'

'I'll only be a minute,' he says.

'Shall I tell that to the child with a broken arm who's been waiting over forty minutes already?' says Chris.

'I'll only be a minute,' Jon Berry repeats.

'Why don't you tell the administration manager or whatever the hell he is called these days that we need a few more computers down here – either that or a few less managers.' With that, Chris turns round to march off and walks slap-bang into the management consultant from Accenture, or wherever. 'And what are *you* doing here?'

'I'm observing,' he replies.

'Observing what? Six people waiting to use a computer? Observing the observer observing someone else, who might actually be doing something if you lot weren't in his way?'

Chris is very obviously about to lose his temper, but he is suddenly distracted by the arrival of a rather dapper-looking member of the rapid response psych team.

'Nigel Andrews!' he exclaims. 'How the very hell are you? I didn't expect to see you down here.'

'Yes, well, I didn't expect to be down here,' says Nigel, a well-kept fiftysomething with thin blond hair that is neatly parted on the right and combed over to the left, attempting to disguise a rather shiny pink bald head. He is wearing a crisp white shirt, a pale patterned silk tie and a very smart, well-cut navy blue suit that whiffs of a prosperous private practice.

'I haven't seen you for . . .' Chris scratches his head. 'Two years?'

'Maybe more.' Nigel nods. 'I'm only doing NHS one day a week now. I simply can't afford to work for you lot much more than that!'

'Really?'

'Yeah. I've moved across, jumped ship.' He then adds in a whisper, like he's announcing a terribly grubby secret, 'I've become a proper shrink. Got a lovely little practice off Wimpole Street where I happily chat to bored housewives about their appalling sex lives. I nod and smile and listen while they tell me about their husbands climbing over them once a week, when what they really prefer is one off the Rampant Rabbit or a whole afternoon sitting on the washing machine. The real problem is, or so they tell me, once you've had rabbit it's hard to go back.' He laughs. 'It's very good to see you. How's Alice?'

'Good, good,' says Chris.

'The children?'

'Good. Caroline is off to Cambridge soon.'

'Really? Medicine?'

'Sadly no. English.'

'Excellent, excellent, she always was clever. Nice girl.' Nigel rubs his hands together, looking round the place, taking in the two SO19 still pacing about. He nods towards the coppers. 'Had a spot of bother earlier, I presume?'

'Just a little shoot-out,' smiles Chris.

'Oh, the joys of the front line!' says Nigel. 'So, right, where's your DSH?'

'Well, good afternoon, Mr Andrews,' I pipe up. 'Shall we go in there' – I point towards Andrea's office – 'and I can talk you through the notes?'

'Good idea,' he says, following me into the office.

David is sitting at Andrea's desk. He looks up and smiles at us. 'Hello. David Smithson, Plastics. Do you need this desk?'

'No, no,' replies Nigel, 'you carry on.'

I sit Nigel down and tell him as much as I know about Katie and her scars and her attempt to kill herself. He listens very intently while picking bits of fluff off his blue trousers. His legs are crossed, right over left, and the right one swings repeatedly. Just as I'm winding up my diagnosis he opens his jacket and pulls out a bottle of pills. He takes two out of the bottle and with a well-practised flick of the head he knocks them straight back without the need for water.

'Bennies,' he says, catching me staring at him. 'It has been a very long day. Is there any coffee around here?'

Two Benzedrine and a cup of coffee is enough to keep even

the most sleep-deprived rock star awake for another couple of hours. With Nigel, the effect appears to be to make him very chatty indeed. By the time Margaret has returned with a coffee with milk and two sugars, Nigel is on a roll. By the time he's finished his cup and is ready to see the patient, it's actually quite hard to get him out of the office.

'I mean the thing is – and you, I'm sure, know this very well, David – most plastic surgery operations could be avoided if they had a bit of therapy first. Take my mate, for example. He's an ENT guy and he had this woman in the other day who had totally unrealistic expectations about the nose job he was about to do. She arrived with her hair grown over her nose, like this big fringe.' He gets out of his chair and starts to imitate the woman. 'And talking to her, he found out that she doesn't go out, because of her nose. She said kids in the street laughed at her, because of her nose, and her whole life was miserable, because of her nose. He then drew back the hair and the nose was totally bloody normal. What she needs is a shrink, not bloody rhinoplasty! She honestly thinks that changing her nose will help her lose four stone, get laid and get a job when in fact all that will happen is that she'll have a new nose!'

'There are some operations that are very effective, actually,' replies David, trying to stick up for his specialism. 'Breast reduction is very good for relieving back pain, for example.'

'Yes, well, maybe,' concedes Nigel. 'But you know that is very specific. In order to get that on the NHS you have to have a BMI of less than twenty-eight per cent and you have to be removing more than five hundred grams off each breast, which is quite a substantial amount of flesh. So you have to be thin with large breasts, which is, let's face it, quite a rare group of women.'

'There's no point in taking big boobs off a fat woman,' says David. 'She'll only see her stomach.'

'True! True!' laughs Nigel, and then gives a little shiver. 'I bet you see bosoms all the time.'

'How did you know?' says David, looking a little shocked.

'You're good-looking and a plastic surgeon. Women must ask you about their breasts all the time.'

'You're right. It drives me mad.'

'Poor you!' I say, rolling my eyes, my heart oh so genuinely bleeding for him. It must be awful to be chased by women who want to bare their breasts to you.

'No, seriously,' says David, his brow furrowing earnestly. 'They're always pulling their tops up and asking what I think of their breasts, and what I want to say is "I think you should put them away." I think they think they are being amusing.'

'Or trying to shock,' says Nigel. 'Get some attention. You should tell them to put them away.'

'No, I should,' he agrees. 'But breast reduction does work, and I suppose to a certain extent so does gender realignment.'

'You say that,' says Nigel. 'But they still have totally un-realistic expectations. I have a mate down the road who works at the best place on the NHS for the whole gender thing.'

David nods in agreement.

'They get the truckers in who want the whole shebang. Noses, vocal cord tightening, the works. Did you know that they have the highest suicide rate? Men wanting gender realignment? Something like seventy per cent if they don't get the op before thirty-five years old. Anyway, my mate, the nose guy, had this hulking great bloke in the other day. He comes in with the dress on, and some photos, with these huge plates of meat for hands, and my mate says, "So, what sort of nose are you looking for?" And the bloke says, "My mates say that I look like Keira Knightley, apparently I have her eyes, so can I have her nose please?" Now *he*, I think, definitely needs a bit more counselling.'

'Yeah, I would agree with that,' says David. 'We were always taught never to operate on a SIMON.'

'A SIMON?' I ask.

'A single immature male obsessive neurotic,' they both reply.

'The outcome is always poor,' David explains. 'They will never be happy regardless of what you do. You are supposed to write down what you have discussed and then you are supposed to get them to sign that they have agreed with what you have discussed so that when they come back six weeks later, kicking up a fuss, you can show them what they agreed to. But, quite frankly, they should be avoided at all costs.'

'I agree,' says Nigel. 'My ENT mate had some bloke come back a few weeks after the op with photos, saying, "This is what I wanted to look like." My friend did suggest that perhaps he might have brought them in before!'

'Well, yes, that is a thought!' I interject. 'Um, shall we go and see Katie? Her mother is also in the waiting room, if you would like to talk to her?'

'Let's do the patient first,' Nigel says, rubbing his hands and getting out of his chair. 'No rest for the wicked.'

I escort him to the cubicle and pull back the curtain to find

Katie in exactly the same position I left her in: lying on her side, facing the wall, the tubes from the IV drip beside her.

'Hi, Katie,' I start. 'I've brought someone along to have a chat with you. To see how you're doing. His name is—'

'Katie, I'm Nigel. I'm here to see how you are and see if anyone can help.' He pulls up a chair. 'Oh dear, oh dear, you look like you've been in the wars. What's happened to you?' His voice is kind and his manner is extremely beguiling. She rolls slightly towards him.

I back away out of the cubicle and leave them to it.

'That your DSH in there?' asks Ian, walking past.

I nod.

'Who's that with her?'

'Some bloke from the psych team called Nigel.'

'Nigel!' Ian grins. 'He's a scream. He hasn't been around for ages. You have to pay two hundred a go to see him now. Hasn't he got some practice on Harley Street?'

'Just off Wimpole Street, I think.'

'He's brilliant. Very good at his job. He worked for the prison service a while back. Counselling murderers. They're either mad, bad or sad, he used to say. I remember him telling me about a man who strangled his girlfriend because she threatened to leave him; transpired that he had also killed something like thirty cats, ripping their heads off in the back garden. Sounded like a lovely bloke.'

'God,' I say, 'that must have been a tough job.'

'No worse than here,' smiles Ian. 'You off today?'

'Yup. Last hour, last shift.'

'What's your next move?'

'Acute Medicine.'

'Good.' He nods. 'A lot less grind than here.'

'Why do you stay?'

'What, here? I love it.' He grins. 'All the shouting, screaming and vomit. My dad was a pub landlord, it makes me feel right at home!'

Ian walks off, with his bag of bloods to deposit down the chute.

I glance over at the empty consultation room; the peonies and chocolates appear to have gone. I feel a terrible pang of guilt. My mouth goes dry and my stomach churns. I wish I had managed to talk properly to June's daughter, Audrey, told her how sorry I was that her mother had died, that she looked like a wonderful person, that she wouldn't have felt that much pain at the end. But then I'm sure Chris said all those things; he is brilliant at that sort of thing. Still, I think I'd like closure of some sort, which is oddly needy of me. I must be tired. Either that or my hangover is creeping up on me.

'Extra special posh chocolate?' asks Andrea, walking through the department with a large open box. 'It is the end of term after all.'

I feel a rush of saliva to my mouth. I'm starving.

'These are extra special, top of the range, I can't think why I'm sharing them with you lot!'

I have my hand poised over the box when I realize that it's Audrey's box. There is no reason why Andrea shouldn't have taken them, they'd only go to waste. Audrey was hardly going to come back to collect them, having identified her mother in the chapel of rest. But even so. My mouth goes completely dry.

'No thank you,' I say.

'Are you sure?' she asks, her plump fingers popping another one into her already full mouth. 'They're very good.'

'Oh, great-looking chocolates,' says Chris, rushing past and picking up two at once. 'Don't mind if I do.' He puts them both in his mouth at the same time. 'Mmm, they are *very* good.'

Back at the far end of the department Jon Berry and his side-kick are finally vacating the area. Well, it is after 5.30 and the end of a very busy day for them, watching other people work. They must be exhausted, in need of a sit-down and a pay rise.

'Ah, good, there you are,' says Nigel, his thinning head of hair poking out between the curtains. 'One quick question.' He drops his voice to a stage whisper. 'If I do need to admit her, is there a bed?'

'Let me check,' I reply.

He smiles and crosses his fingers at me. I walk to the wall phone just by the computer and spend the next twenty minutes trying to call the psych ward to see if they have any beds. The amount of time I have wasted doing this in my career doesn't bear thinking about. You call and call and no one ever picks up, and then suddenly you find the line is engaged. Is someone actually finally picking up? Or is it just another sod like you calling in the hope that someone answers? And then, just when you think you might brave the walk up there, some grumpy arse answers the thing and all you want to do is shout your head off about how pissed off you are to have been kept waiting, except you don't because you want them to find you an empty hospital bed, which as we all know is as rare as rocking-horse shit.

'Oh, hello!' I blurt, stifling my desire to shout down the phone. 'We have a very vulnerable woman in A&E . . .'

I explain Katie's case and say that we are waiting for a report from the psych team, at which they nearly hang up. It's only after another few minutes of grovelling that they allow me to call back on another number and intimate that if I am very lucky they might have something.

As I hang up, Nigel comes up the corridor towards me. 'So,' he says, nodding his head towards Andrea's office, 'in here?'

I sit and listen as he ticks off Katie's long list of problems on his fingers. Anorexia, OCD, low self-esteem, amphetamine and laxatives abuse, and more than likely some sort of abuse at home too, either from the father or the mother, he wasn't sure. Either way he would prefer it if she were kept in and monitored for a while, and she seems willing.

'So there is no need for sectioning,' he concludes.

'Who are you putting away now?' asks Ian, coming into the office with a broad grin on his face. 'How are you, me old fruit?'

Nigel stands and he and Ian hug, slapping each other heartily on the back.

'All the better for seeing you!' says Nigel. 'I can't believe you're still here. Been passed over again?'

'Ha bloody ha! Seen any more lunchtime fanny recently?'

'God, I'd forgotten that!' He laughs, his eyes rolling. Then he looks at me. 'It's not what you're thinking.'

'I wasn't thinking anything,' I say.

'You were.'

I *was* thinking something, but perhaps not what he thought I was thinking.

'I was supervising shrink for this fellow shrink,' Nigel explains, 'who came to me saying he had a problem. He had this client who had come in dressed in pigtails and a short skirt, talking like Minnie Mouse, and then a week later she had come back with a skirt so short you could see her arse in reception, and then when she got into his office she had opened her legs and done the full Sharon Stone. So I asked him what he did and he said that he had said to the woman, "I'm terribly sorry but I can see your vagina, do you want to talk about that?" To which she apparently hit the roof and accused him of touching her.'

'Oh God,' I say.

'The shrink's worst nightmare,' he agrees. 'I mean, he hadn't handled it very well. He hadn't talked about his home life enough, or used the word "we" to indicate that he had a partner. Fortunately his practice nurse vouched for him in the end.'

'And there was the small fact that he batted for my team,' says Ian.

'That's true,' concurs Nigel.

'So, how's everything?' asks Ian, rubbing his hands.

'Oh, I've got this great case at the moment,' says Nigel. 'A man who gets an erection every time a woman sneezes. And then he has to follow her and rub himself up against her. It has got so bad that he's in danger of losing his job.'

'No shit,' says Ian.

'Well, I know. He has become so obsessed that it now takes him hours to get to work. He will get on the Tube in the morning and start doing his sums. He has worked out there are more women on the platform than there are in the carriage, that he is statistically more likely to hear a sneeze there. So what happens is that he travels from station to station and gets off every time he can see more women. So it takes him hours to get to work. His wife is very understanding.'

'His wife!' laughs Ian.

'I know,' Nigel nods. 'It's a hard case to crack, and it's getting worse. I blame Nanny, I think. Perhaps he was sitting very close to his nanny when he was tiny and then she sneezed and he sexualized it. If he hears a woman sneeze in a shop, that's it. He can be there all day.'

'He needs to marry someone with nympho hay fever,' I suggest.

'Good idea,' Nigel agrees.

'And how's your klepto lawyer?' asks Ian.

'Oh.' His face becomes serious. 'Now that is a disaster.' He looks at me again. 'I was looking after a lawyer with a rather bad shoplifting problem and it was progressively getting worse. Anyway, my colleague and I decided that it was something to do with repressed sexuality, and she finally admitted that she hadn't had an orgasm for a decade or so. So she was reintroduced to masturbation at the age of fifty-four and we thought that she was doing very well until she was arrested on a double yellow line masturbating in her car outside Marks and Spencer with her pockets full of smoked salmon.

She had done the lifting and then been so overcome with desire that she couldn't control herself.'

'She wasn't muttering "This isn't just a wank, this is a Marks and Spencer wank," was she?' asks Ian, half-closing his eyes and frotting himself off.

'Excuse me,' says Andrea, looking from the wanking consultant to the sniggering plastic surgeon to the giggling psychiatrist and then to me, 'I have a phone call for you.'

'Me?' I ask.

'Yes,' she sighs with irritation. 'They have a bed for you upstairs.'

6–7 p.m.

Nigel sits in Andrea's office regaling Ian and David with more of his stories while I try to concentrate on sorting out Katie's paperwork. I go back out into the waiting room to see if I can have a calm and reasonable chat with Katie's mother, who is firmly ensconced in the far corner next to the television, leafing through *Now* magazine. She seems remarkably relaxed for someone whose daughter has just tried to kill herself. But then, it is extraordinary how different people deal with stress. I once treated a woman whose only way of coping with anything too tricky was to fall asleep. She had stress-induced narcolepsy, and every time she was put under pressure, she would keel over. In the end she was put on heavy-duty beta-blockers so nothing really touched her again.

'Good evening, Mrs Heywood,' I begin with Katie's mother.

Her thin, pinched face looks up from studying Cheryl Cole's fashion tips.

'Katie's fine,' I say quickly, to reassure her. 'But we would like to keep her in, you know, just to make sure.'

'OK then,' she says. Her grey eyes are impassive.

'She may be in for a couple of days.'

'Do you need me to sign anything?' she asks.

'Katie's not a minor so she can sign her own forms,' I reply. 'But I'm sure she would like to see you now. I'll find out where she's going to be so you can come and see her. Visiting hours are four p.m. till eight p.m. You could pop in and see her now if you like. She might also need some stuff. A toothbrush, that sort of thing.'

'No,' she says, her nose curling, like she has smelt something bad, 'you're all right.' She gets up. 'I've got stuff to do. She can send me a text later if she wants.'

'Oh, right.'

I'm not really sure what to do. Try and persuade her to see her daughter, even if that causes more aggro, or just let her go? Atrophied by indecision, I watch her leave. She slopes off, staring at the floor, her shoulders hunched. She's got the walk of a depressive. I remember talking to a psychiatrist once about depression and she told me that you can always tell a lot about people from their walk. The body has a rhythm, and the way you swing your arms and the balance and motion of your gait can indicate so many things, from depression to the early onset of Parkinson's. Depressives rarely look up, towards the sky. In fact one of the suggested therapies for depression is to walk, to get the blood circulating, and look up at the clouds. Movement releases endorphins that help improve your mood. But from the way Katie's mother is walking, she's not seen the sun or the clouds for months. I'm willing to bet that she would benefit from a bit of therapy herself.

I look around, and the waiting room is seriously beginning to fill up now. There are a few cuts that need stitching, what looks like a dog bite, a broken wrist, some bloke who's been hit in the face. There are a couple of elderly people sitting in the corner, and one woman who is pacing around tugging at her clothes, looking a little delirious – suffering, I'd say, from an untreated kidney infection. The bins are overflowing, there's rubbish on the floor, the water-cooler is empty, and the spotty teen on reception is not coping well with the queue of people waiting to be registered. So far so normal. This is the 'going home from work' crowd, the slips, the bumps, the scrapes. Soon we'll get the cooking-dinner injuries, the burns and cuts. And then the drinking begins.

But I'm very nearly out of here. I feel my mood lift as I go back through the swing doors.

Nigel is still talking. Clearly his bennies are working a treat.

'But they're not always nutters, you know,' he declares. 'Sometimes you have to take their stories seriously.'

'Yeah, right,' laughs Ian.

'No, seriously. I had a mate who was working at Barnet hospital when this bloke came in insisting that he had been poisoned. They didn't listen, obviously, they told him he had diarrhoea, but he kept on insisting. He did look very unwell so they kept him in, but all that happened was the diarrhoea and vomiting. They tried to grow cultures with his stools but nothing happened. There was no bacteria, which was odd, and the bloke was getting worse. By the next morning my mate, the consultant, came in so the guy asked him, "Are you the senior man here?" To which he replied "Yes," and the patient asked if he could have a private word. So they disappeared into a side office where the patient suddenly announced that he used to be an agent, that he was once a KGB officer, and now the KGB were after him, they had tried to poison him, and my friend *must* help him. My friend of course agreed and immediately went off and called the psych team. It wasn't until a black Merc started circling the building and some blokes in dark suits from the Home Office turned up that they started to believe him. Hilarious, don't you think?'

'So who was he?' asks David, leaning forward over his desk.

'Alexander Litvinenko!' answers Nigel, slightly incredulously.

David looks blank.

'The Russian spy who died of polonium poisoning?'

'Oh, right, him,' he nods. 'I remember that. A bit.'

Before anyone has time to berate David for his extra-ordinarily crap memory, Louise pops her head round the office door.

'Oh, hi, there you are,' she says to me. 'Um, I just wanted to say goodbye, and good luck, and thank you for your help today.'

'That's OK.' I smile. 'Are you off?'

'Yup,' she says, with a small shrug. 'See you around . . . I guess.'

'Yeah,' I say, still smiling. 'It's been great to work with you. You're a wonderful doctor. You're going to go far.'

'Well, as far as St Thomas's!'

167

'Oh great, I'm glad I've got you both here,' says Chris, marching into the office.

We both turn and face him. I'm expecting a little pep talk, wishing us good luck in all that we do, and hoping we'll remember them when Louise is the foxiest of Max Foxes around, reconstructing faces from small bits of thigh, and I am literally raising the dead as King of Acute Medicine, or a master heart surgeon. Either way I am grand and brilliant. I can also see Louise's feathers fluff up, waiting for her plaudits.

'Excellent, great,' says Chris. 'OK . . . so . . . one of you has to work a double shift tonight.'

'What?' says Louise.

'We are three down and we only have a locum covering for the SHOs.' His eyes dart from me to Louise and back again. He looks a little sweaty, to say the least. 'You do the graveyard shift and I promise you can leave at three a.m. It's nothing you haven't done before.'

'We're not supposed to have to do this,' says Louise, all irritated. 'Isn't that what the European Working Time Directive is for?'

'Yes, well, tell that to the locum who I know has already done a shift down at St Joseph's, as that's where he works normally, and tell that to all the presentations who are planning to pop in tonight with only four doctors manning the place. I know it's all-change bloody Tuesday, but for three bloody doctors to call in sick – and I use that term loosely – is bloody unforgivable.'

'Well, I've got a barbecue to go to,' declares Louise.

'A barbecue?' Chris looks incredulous.

'It's my sister's birthday,' she says, a sweet smile spreading across her pretty face. 'Her twenty-sixth,' she adds, trying to give a little more significance to the event.

I look at Chris for a reaction. If he is having sex with her, he's hiding it pretty well. All I can see on his face is irritation and a growing desire to lose his rag.

'I'll do it,' I say.

'You will?' both Louise and Chris ask at the same time.

'Why not?' I say.

I'd rather not, of course, but I only have an evening of Emma's rather poor cooking and repeats of *Location, Location, Location* to look forward to, so why the hell not? It also means I get to miss the first day on Acute Medicine down the road, which is a joy. There's nothing worse than watching half a hospital wandering around looking for the toilets. I've done it a few times now and, let me tell you, it is painful. The patients' charts don't get read, the wrong drugs are shelled out in the wrong amounts, and no one knows the entrance codes to the theatres, the drugs cabinets, or even how you sign on at the computer. I'd much rather sit out that chaos watching Holly and Phillip on *This Morning* with a lapful of toast and Marmite.

'I'll phone through to your consultant and tell him you've done an emergency double and to give you tomorrow off,' says Chris, like he's reading my mind.

'Perfect,' I say.

'Thank you,' says Louise, looking grateful. 'I can't bear that graveyard shift.'

'It's fine,' I say. 'It's August and half the population are on holiday. What's the worst that can happen?'

There really shouldn't be any need for me to pull a double shift tonight, and technically I'm not allowed to, but it does still happen. Although the days when we came to work on Friday and didn't leave till Monday are over, they will stand me in good stead tonight. I will be on call, so to speak, and I'll be given a bed somewhere in the hospital; whether or not I get to lie down on it is a different matter. I am technically supposed to be on a forty-eight-hour week, which basically means that some doctors have become expert shift workers who watch the clock and walk straight out of the building as soon as their hours are up. Gone are the days when you would catheterize yourself just to get through an operation. Now doctors leave halfway through cases, midway through consultations, which means patients going into an operation only to have someone totally different meet them when they come round. There is no longer any continuity of care. Patients are handed on from one doctor to another, with all the nuances of individual treatment lost in transit.

Consultants now have productivity-related pay. They are paid, like celebrities, per PA, or personal appearance. You can negotiate anything between nine and twelve PAs a week with the hospital, which means that those who are rewarded the most are those who play the system the best.

And still we have to do double shifts, and still locum doctors turn up who have already done eleven hours somewhere else before clocking on here. I used to think some of them were workshy tosspots when I caught them catnapping on the coats in the common room, but then you realize they've done eleven hours somewhere else and you forgive them a ten-minute lie-down every so often. I remember being so tired that I used to nod off during my own case presentations. I'd be standing at the whiteboard telling my fellow doctors about how I had managed to spot the signs of malaria, then fall into a snooze, only to come round having drawn a big red line over my chart. But, as I said, at least I am well practised at functioning on fewer than five hours, sleep over a weekend, so tonight won't be too much of a drag. I only pray that we are busy. It sounds mad, I know, but the busier A&E is, the less time I'll have to think and the less time I'll have to realize quite how tired I am.

'Really, thank you for doing this,' says Louise, giving my shoulder a squeeze.

I have to admit I was hoping for a slightly more generous gesture. Not quite along the lines of Margaret and Steve this morning, but something a little more expansive. A peck on the cheek?

'That's OK,' I shrug.

'No, I mean it,' she says. 'It's very kind of you. And good luck for next year.'

She leans in to hug me. Better than nothing I suppose.

'I'm sure we'll see each other around.'

'Yep,' I say. 'Good luck to you too.'

Not that she needs it, of course. She is pretty and clever, the sort of woman men like me do double shifts for. She's not going to run into many difficulties. I am on the verge of asking her for her phone number, but I realize it's a pointless exercise. I am never going to have the balls to call her, and Louise is never going to call me.

'See you around,' I add, lamely.

She smiles lamely back and heads out of the office, off to her sister's birthday barbecue.

Back out in the hall, the locum has turned up. He has dark curly hair and a winning smile.

'Hi,' he says, coming over to shake my hand. 'Ben. I think I've worked with you before.'

'Oh, right,' I say, searching through my raddled old hungover memory for his name or face.

'A couple of months back?' he says.

'Right, I remember,' I lie.

'This is my last locum shift,' he says. 'I'm joining a private plastics firm next week. I didn't get my consultancy – again.' He rolls his eyes, then moves over to the sterile gel dispenser to clean his hands.

'That's annoying,' I say.

'It's more than annoying,' he asserts. 'I did a super specialism in rhinology last year so that I could, you know, make myself more attractive, and I was reduced to A&E shifts to make some cash, and now . . .' He sighs. 'Now I'm going to have to listen to people bang on about why they don't like their noses at a hundred and fifty for a half-hour whine, when I used to do fifteen patients in three hours at Guy's. But, you know, what doesn't kill you . . .'

Ben is one of the growing number of limbo doctors: all qualified but nowhere to go. While many of them earn money doing locum shifts, waiting for a job to come through, others are leaving the NHS to set up in the world of extreme beauty. The world of Botox, collagen and fillers used to be the remit of the beautician with a needle fetish. Rather scarily, anyone with a rudimentary knowledge of eyeliner and Chanel's new spring/summer colours was allowed to inject anyone else, just so long as they signed a consent form. But these days extremely talented surgeons who were once reconstructing faces after car crashes are now finding themselves washed up on the high street. So the NHS's loss is the WAG's gain. Who better to pump your face full of Sculptra than someone who actually knows what goes on below the skin?

'There are a few perks for pumping carp lips all day though,' Ben grins. 'My mate, who owns the practice, says he's being offered blow jobs all the time.'

'What?' Two minutes of talking to Ben and already un-employment is sounding a little rosier.

'Oh yeah,' he nods. 'Blow jobs for Botox. Sex for surgery. It's all going on. He says it happens at least once a week. It's mainly the Essex girls and the Russians. They're twenty-one and they come in and start to rub your cock when you're standing over them with the needle. Or they rub your hand over their boobs, or run their fingers up and down your thigh.'

'And does he? You know, shag them?'

'Sometimes, but you don't want to get yourself a reputation as a place where you can do that. Otherwise you would be inundated. Imagine how many call-girls get Botox. He'd end up running a knocking shop. But I know he's done it. Also, you have to be so careful as they can always accuse you of stuff. He has an assistant in there with him, to cover him in case of any difficult behaviour, but the girls always find a way of getting rid of her, asking her for some water, to get their handbag that they have "left" in reception.' He does the quotation thing in the air with his fingers. 'There were two girls in a few weeks back, Russian—'

'He does two patients at a time?'

'Oh yeah, mothers and daughters, mates on a trip up to town. It's only Botox and collagen for Chrissake.'

'True.'

'Anyway, these Russians came in and started talking between themselves about giving him a blow job and having a threesome with him. Little did they know that he did French and Russian at university before going on to do medicine so he understood every word.'

'That must have perked up his day no end.'

'Yes, well, the other day was a little different. He had this gay bloke in for liposuction. He was doing the gut and the moobs using a local anaesthetic. And while he was sucking away with a probe in one hand, the aspirator in the other, the bloke's hand crept up underneath the green sheet and grabbed his cock.'

My mouth opens in shock.

'Yup,' continues Ben, grinning back at me. 'So there he is, with both his hands occupied and someone else's vice-like grip on his genitals. He can't do anything. If he stops the op the man will just deny it, he'll lose the six grand for the operation and it will be his word against the patient, and the patient will deny all knowledge, and he'll probably have to do the op again anyway. Or he can just carry on. The nurses could see what was happening and refused to help him out in any way, shape or form. They just watched his eyes gently water over the mask as he looked longingly at them for help!'

I'm laughing quite loudly now.

'So my mate had his cock and balls cupped for twenty minutes while he sucked as much fat out of the man's stomach as possible. It was the quickest op he's ever done!'

'I bet, I bet!' I laugh. 'So that's where you're going after this?'

'Absolutely,' he smiles. 'Think how much more you can charge for your acid peel if it's administered by a doctor.'

'Double?' I suggest.

'And the rest!' He winks.

I follow Ben towards the computer. I haven't laughed this much for ages. It makes such a difference who you work with in this business. I have a feeling this shift might fly by.

Suddenly the swing doors slam open and a gurney speeds in with three paramedics steaming along beside it.

'Stabbing!' barks one of the green jumpsuits.

'Stabbing!' echoes another. 'Suspected punctured lung, possible punctured heart and left pulmonary artery!'

'Stabbing!' Chris shouts up at me. 'Get yourself down here, *now*!'

The next five minutes are hellish. Turns out this sixteen-year-old boy was stabbed through the heart as he got off the bus at his stop, on his way back from football practice. He'd looked at someone 'funny', or so the story goes. So the other bloke's mate stuck a six-inch blade through his chest, at least twice, possibly three times. It took about seven minutes for the ambulance to arrive, and in that time he picked up an entourage. With the victim comes his mother, two sisters, an aunt, their mates and about another six or seven interested parties. A&E is packed. There's shouting, there's screaming. His mother keeps shoving her head into the cubicle, beseeching us to keep her son alive.

Despite his black skin, the boy is white. Literally all the colour is draining from his face. There is blood on the floor, blood on the table, a trail of blood all the way up the corridor and back through the double doors. It is pouring out of him. Andrea and Margaret have set up IVs of O neg but it seems to be bubbling straight through him and back out on to the floor. We are skidding and slipping in the stuff. Chris cuts open his chest and both of us stare inside, trying to work out what has happened. It is gory and cut up in there; it is impossible to work out where to start. His young heart is madly pumping away, but it's running out of blood to pump. His blood pressure is plummeting. His mother is screaming, his sisters are wailing, and Chris and I are desperately searching through the pools of blood and severed pipes trying to work out which ones to try and stem.

'Here,' says Chris.

'No, here,' I suggest.

'Oh fucking hell,' he says.

The pumping heart suddenly ceases. The monitor goes monotone and there is a wild scream from the other side of the curtains. I look at Chris. He is covered in sweat and blood; he looks like a slaughterman after a hard day's cull. He stares back at me. I am up to my elbows in blood. His expression is desperate. His eyes are hollow. But there is nothing we can do. Nothing.

'Please can you call it?' he asks.

7–8 p.m.

It was all over in twenty minutes. From the first slam of the double doors to the horrible sound of the heart monitor flat-lining; it took no time at all. He was alive, struggling for his life. And then minutes later he's dead. I think it's the chaos, or the fact that your heart is beating nineteen to the dozen, that makes it appear longer, that makes you feel like you are living three lifetimes in those few short minutes.

But of course the fallout is huge. The family are in-consolable. They want responses to questions no one has answers to. Their son/brother was not in a gang. He was on his way back from football. He was two minutes from his own front door. It's always the nice ones who get it. The ones who were minding their own business. He did not carry and was not carrying a knife. Although you can hardly blame any of them for carrying knives. It is part of the culture. It's very hard being a teenage boy in the shitty areas of this city. You get picked on on your way to school and again on the way back. You have to carry a knife for your own protection. Or at least that is what they think. The results of which we see time and time again.

I have stitched up so many young men here who have been knifed while attacking someone or who have been wounded in self-defence, I have ceased to judge who was in the right and who was in the wrong. I tell you, the temptation to do a bad job on some psychotic shit who has brought two other victims in here with him is high. But in the end you do a professional job, because you are a professional; though I might just use a little less painkiller or a slightly thicker needle than usual. But it will all look more or less the same.

Chris and Andrea are dealing with the boy's parents. His mother is wailing so loudly, her grief is so palpable, that they have closed the office door. No number of cups of sweet tea and biscuits from the Fox's box that are specially reserved for patients' relatives is going to calm her down. I can see Chris holding her hand, patting it, stroking, trying to calm her down. She eventually collapses sobbing on his shoulder, and Chris pats her arm.

Eventually the police arrive, all four of them with pens poised, trying to work out how it all happened so quickly and so tragically, in broad daylight, on a dull evening in August. Finally the family release Chris, and are taken somewhere more private for the questions, the recriminations and the what-ifs to begin. The blood is mopped up and the boy's body is wheeled off to the morgue.

Ben comes up to me in the corridor and taps me on the

178

shoulder. 'Have you seen a nurse?' he asks. 'My PFO in here needs stitches.'

I check my watch; it's not even seven thirty. 'That's a bit early for a PFO, isn't it?'

'Office party,' he says.

The pissed-and-fell-over presentations don't usually start arriving until after nine p.m. You have to give them enough time to get steaming drunk after work, and three hours of solid boozing usually does the trick. Obviously on 'special occasions' such as England football matches, during the Christmas party season, on St Patrick's Day or even just on a plain old bank holiday, they can come in earlier. But more usually people tend to wait until nineish before falling down the stairs and breaking their faces, or tripping off the pavement and breaking their legs. This bloke, according to Ben, has slipped over in a pool of Pimm's on a lino floor and cut his forehead open. It's not serious. It requires about six stitches.

Most of the nurses have changed shift now. Andrea is still here, briefing the fresh batch on what's been going down in here today. I am just about to be a little pissed off that Margaret hasn't bothered to say goodbye when I spot her coming towards me in her navy blue coat.

'It's a little hot for that, isn't it?' I say, looking at her coat.

'It's practically autumn,' she smiles. 'Anyway, you never know what the weather is doing in here. We don't see daylight for twelve hours at a time.'

'True,' I say. 'You off then?'

'Yup,' she says. 'I'm having dinner with Steve.'

'Really?'

'Well, you know, he's off tomorrow and, you know, he's got his girlfriend Alicia . . .'

'I see.'

'Our last chance,' she says. 'Bye then.' She gives me a kiss on the cheek.

She looks much younger out of her sky-blue cotton/polyester-mix tunic. The flowered dress poking out from underneath her coat makes her look much more girlie and sweet. I can only hope that Steve knows what he is doing. I am not sure Margaret is as Teflon-coated as he thinks she is.

'I'll come by and see you when I'm over in this neck of the woods,' I say.

'Yeah, you won't,' she says. 'Don't worry, we're used to you doctors coming and going and leaving us behind.'

'Well, I hope to see you one day.' I smile, and kiss her back. 'Bye, Margaret.'

'Bye,' she says, with a little wave. 'Tell Steve not to be too long. I'm waiting in the Prince of Wales opposite.'

Steve is clocking off at eight tonight, the lucky bastard. Hopefully we will be joined by another SHO at the end of their rotation, plus another senior consultant at least, to join Ian, as Chris is about to leave as well. Things generally kick off from here on until about two a.m., so we usually have a minimum of a couple of consultants on call, to tide us over the tricky bit. But at this time of year, with everyone moving tomorrow, any sort of shit can happen.

'Great, you!' says Ian. 'Come with me. I've just been bleeped. We've got a heart attack coming in due to anaphylactic shock. Some dental nurse has eaten a peanut.'

'Resus two?' I ask, trotting on after him.

'Good. We want adrenalin, atropine, the whole fucking medicine cabinet. She is twenty-three years old, let's try not to lose her.'

The whole of A&E springs into action. Andrea's ample bosom comes undulating towards me beneath her midnight-blue uniform. Stacy, a nurse who I have worked with many times before, rushes over with IV stands, and Connie is whisking all the monitors into place. Chris is standing to attention despite the fact that he was on his way out, and we are all staring at the double door in tense anticipation.

The doors slam open; the trolley comes speeding in, with two paramedics running either side of it.

'In here, in here!' shouts Ian, waving his hands.

They rush the trolley into Resus 2 and everyone sets to work. This is a well-practised, well-run manoeuvre. There really is nothing like the NHS when it comes to an acute emergency like a heart attack. We are a well-oiled crash team, and everyone knows the drill. All the drugs and equipment are on tap.

On goes a new oxygen mask, on goes the heart monitor, in go the IV tubes. It's like clockwork.

'Any knowledge of any ops?' Ian asks the paramedics.

'Not that we know of,' one of them replies.

'Administering clot-busters,' announces Ian. 'Let's hope no one's cut her open in the last couple of weeks.'

I look at the dental nurse. Her face is drained of colour, her skin is covered in sweat, her stats are looking poor on the monitor, and she's a big girl. Her BMI must be over 40. It's not looking good for her, despite the fact that she's in her early twenties. But we have all done this before, so no one is rushing and no one is panicking.

'Adrenalin,' announces Stacy, approaching with a large syringe and an even larger needle.

'In the heart,' says Ian, looking at the girl's stats.

'The heart?' checks Stacy. 'Really?'

'We don't want to lose her. D'you hear?' says Chris.

'But the heart?'

'Straight into the heart,' both Ian and Chris say at the same time.

'OK,' I say. I take the syringe and spritz some liquid out of the end to make sure there are no bubbles. 'Here goes.' I plunge the needle into her sternum, avoiding the large expanse of bosom, and aim for the heart. I inject the transparent liquid and pull quickly out.

We all stand back, waiting for the drugs to kick in. But instead of her system rebooting, she flatlines.

'Shit! Fuck! Defibrillator!'

Stacy rushes the machine forward.

'Stand back!' continues Ian, holding the panels aloft, waiting for them to clear. 'Clear!'

He shocks the girl. Her whole body spasms off the trolley. And then relaxes back down again. We all look at the monitor. Nothing.

'Clear!' commands Ian.

He shocks her again. Still nothing.

'Clear!' he says again.

The dental nurse's back arches up and falls back down again. Again nothing.

'Massage!' Ian shouts at me.

I leap on her chest and start pounding it with my fists, trying to get her heart moving.

'Keep going! More adrenalin!'

I leap off as Ian injects another huge jab of liquid into her IV. We all fall silent and stare at the monitor. Hoping for a beep, a sign that there is still hope. Nothing.

'OK then, clear!' shouts Ian.

He has the paddles in the air; he barely waits for us to move. *Bang.* Her body lifts off the table and collapses down. The monotone hum continues.

'Clear!'

Nothing.

'Clear!'

Nothing.

'Clear!'

Nothing.

'Adrenalin!'

This goes on and on and on. None of us wants to lose her. She's twenty-three, for Chrissake. We've had one youngster die in here already today, no one wants another. We carry on with the paddles and the massage. We are supposed to wait two minutes between each shock and administer constant CPR, but we don't. Ian is desperate to restart her heart. I am desperate to restart her heart. We are all bloody desperate. For ten, fifteen minutes we shock, massage and hope.

'I think I am going to call it,' says Chris.

'Just a bit longer,' says Ian, sweat pouring down the side of his face.

'No, no, that's it,' says Chris, shaking his head. 'Nineteen forty-three. Well done, Ian. You tried your best. We gave it our all, there was nothing else we could have done. Really, team, honestly, nothing else we could have done. Poor girl . . .'

We all stand and stare, sweating, shattered. Open-mouthed. How did that happen so quickly? What a huge shock. And the girl is so young.

'You did what you could,' Chris continues. 'We all did what we could . . .'

None of us can move. My heart is pounding in my chest. My limbs feel like lead. We all carry on standing there. No one moves. No one says anything.

'Can someone look through her pockets and see if she has a donor card,' asks Chris finally, interrupting the exhausted silence. 'Are her parents here? We need to persuade them of the merits of transplant.'

Organ donation is one of the more controversial areas of our job. The problem is that the number of people wanting organs is on the increase, whereas the number of people donating is not. We currently have about ten thousand patients awaiting transplants in the UK with three people a day dying while still waiting. We don't have an opt-out donor policy in this country where you are considered onboard unless you state otherwise, so one of the more unpleasant aspects of our job is to persuade grieving parents or loved ones to sign a donor form, while the patient is still useful. Obviously the longer we wait the less useful the body is.

There are three ways of donating. Heart-beating donation, where the patient is dead but the heart is still working and oxygenating the blood, making the transplant much more likely to succeed. This is often the case with brain-damaged patients. Or there is non-heart-beating donation where the patient is dead, from a heart attack for instance, and the heart has stopped working. Speed is of the essence here, as the longer we wait the more the organ quality deteriorates. Then there is live-organ donation – kidneys and bone marrow, that sort of thing. They are usually donated by relatives and siblings. Occasionally some extremely altruistic donor will donate to someone they don't know, but this is rare.

With such a huge demand for organs and so few donors, there is also of course an illegal worldwide trade in organs. The kidney market dominates this trade in body parts, as they are in greatest demand and are easiest to harvest and transport. According to the World Health Organisation, of the seventy thousand or so kidney transplants that take place worldwide, some 20 per cent, perhaps up to fifteen thousand kidneys, could be trafficked. China, India, Pakistan, Egypt, Brazil, the Philippines, Moldova and Romania are among the leading providers of trafficked organs, which are exported to the US, Europe, the United Arab Emirates, Saudi Arabia and especially Israel. This is tantamount to a body tax on the very poor for the benefit of the rich. Kidneys go for around £75,000, with the donor getting between £1,500 and £7,000 for their kidney; the rest is paid to the traffickers. But when the average waiting time for a kidney in the US is ten years and most dialysis patients die within half that time, you can see why there is an ask-no-questions policy operating in some of their less scrupulous hospitals. But when you hear the stories of Indian women being forced to sell a kidney to provide a dowry for their daughters, or children growing up in the Third World being offered lock, stock and barrel to the highest bidder, it makes it more important to sign a donor card. It's hard to ascertain how many trafficked organs are transplanted here in the UK. All I know is that the number will be increasing rather than diminishing.

Stacy very sweetly volunteers to go with Chris to ask the girl's parents, who are sitting in Andrea's office. It is not something I have found easy to do in the past. So sorry your daughter's dead, do you mind if we carve her up? We have all been on this course that basically teaches us how to ask nicely and not cause offence. But all the same, it's extremely difficult.

Ian is standing next to the dead girl filling in the relevant post-death forms and Andrea is pulling out tubes and unplugging all the machines when Stacy comes back.

'That was quick,' says Ian.

'The answer's yes,' says Stacy. 'Apparently she has always said that is what she wants to do.'

'Great, well done.' Ian slaps her on the back. 'Good job.'

'I know, I'm amazed. I was prepared for so much more back-chat.'

'Well, well done, you've made some very ill people very happy.'

'Yeah, I'm thrilled.'

Just then the heart monitor beeps. We stop what we are doing. It beeps again. We all stare.

'What are you doing to the machine?' asks Ian, in a slow and quiet voice.

'Nothing,' replies Andrea.

'Really nothing?' asks Ian. 'Because this is not a good time to crack a joke.'

'Yes, really nothing,' she replies.

There is a loud rasping sound as the corpse inhales a huge gulp of air and then coughs.

'Jesus fuck!' gasps Ian. 'Stacy, run along and tell Mr and Mrs Whatever-their-name-is that their daughter is still alive!'

8–9 p.m.

To say that we are surprised by the Lazarus-like resurrection of Gabriella Turner is an understatement. Ian is fairly mortified, but the person who is the most embarrassed is Chris. It's not often that he calls a death only for the person to wake up a few minutes later.

Amazingly, resurrections are not as rare as you might think. We get one or two a year. The drugs we use are so goddamn strong these days that it takes a fairly determined heart to die. But they can also take a bit of time to react. I can't help but think that in Gabriella's case it was the second jab of adrenalin that launched her back into the land of the living. Sadly, the transplant team will be a little put out. Chris was straight on the phone to them when Gabriella came back. And apart from getting their hopes up, we also look like a right bunch of knob-end idiots who can't tell the dead from the living. I imagine the joke will be around the hospital by tomorrow morning. Fortunately I won't be here to take the rap.

I remember when I was just out of training nearly four years ago and I was working up near Manchester. We had a woman come in who'd had a head trauma, which had left her with part of her brain coming out of her ear. The surgeon basically wrote her off. I mean, you would, wouldn't you? Who can survive with a bit of brain seeping out of their head? So we lined her up for a total organ transplant. Even her corneas were pledged to someone. Anyway, in the end we removed the bit of brain from her ear, and she lived! She didn't just pull through, she was totally fine, and everyone had to stand down. No one was best pleased with the surgeon. Fortunately I was so far down the pecking order that no one remembered me even being there. The surgeon got the piss taken out of him for months after that.

But it is rare for a patient to come out of something like this unscathed. You can't have that much downtime and expect to emerge the other side with all five senses intact. You never know though. There are always exceptions. Maybe Gabriella is one of those.

Her parents crowd into the cubicle to witness their daughter's miraculous recovery for themselves. Her large, big-chested mother weeps; her father just keeps shaking his head like he can't quite believe it; the younger brother stands around in the background, his mouth open, catching flies.

'I think I need a cigarette,' I say to no one in particular.

'I'll come with you,' says Ben.

'How about your PFO?'

'He's being stitched,' he says. 'I've let one of the shiny new students loose on him.' He shrugs. 'He's pissed, he won't notice a thing.'

'True,' I say, glad of the company. 'Come this way.'

Outside in the fresh air I feel a little better. I hadn't realized quite how exhausted I was until I met with the real world. The sky is that glorious pale fresh blue it turns immediately after a sunset. It will be dark soon and the city will start to unleash its shadowy secrets upon us. We always get the weirdest, saddest things during the night-shift. There are some presentations that only come out after dark.

'You again,' says Mary, walking towards me in her coat.

'Ditto,' I say. I do the introductions with Ben. 'I thought you were out for the day.'

'I came back to check on Marsha,' she says, lighting up a menthol cigarette.

'That's nice of you.'

'Well, she's only fifteen and I only live around the corner.' She smiles. 'You can't keep me away from here.'

'You been here long?' asks Ben, very much giving her the once-over.

'A couple of years,' she replies. 'I used to be a legal secretary.'

'Really?' he says.

'Then I retrained. I wanted to do something more worthwhile.'

'Didn't we all,' I say.

'And you liked babies,' adds Ben.

'People,' she corrects. 'I spend most of my time talking to the mothers. Particularly when they are in labour. What else are you supposed to do, sitting there for hours at a time?'

'How is Marsha?' I ask.

'She seems OK. The father has gone, pending a DNA test. But baby Destiny is well.'

'Good.' I nod. 'It's nice to hear some good news for a change.'

'Oh,' says Ben, scratching his groin. 'While you're here. Would you mind checking out my genital warts?'

'What?' Mary almost chokes on her fag.

'My warts,' he says. 'The midwives at St Joseph's do it all the time.'

'Just because I look up fannies all day doesn't mean I'm happy to look at your genitals,' Mary says. 'Check out your own warts. You're a doctor, aren't you?'

'True. But I'm not a bloody gymnast. Do you honestly think that if a man could properly examine his own penis he would ever go out to work?'

'I am not going anywhere near your cock,' she says, putting her hands in the air.

'Mate?' Ben says, turning to me with a pleading look in his eyes. 'They're very painful.'

'Fuck off,' I say, throwing my fag across the car park. 'Have you got a mint?' I ask Mary.

'Of course,' she says, rooting around in her pocket. 'Are you on all night?'

I chat briefly to Mary before returning to A&E. She's a nice girl, with a feisty attitude; ironically for Ben, I think she lives with one of the STD doctors attached to Maternity. I remember her telling me once you could always tell when the university students were back in town or there had been a particularly festive freshers week as the STD doctors were rushed off their feet. The tropical disease department also always gets a surge at the beginning of term. Sex and travel – God, I'd love to go back to being a student again. Life was so much simpler then.

Back in A&E I find that Andrea has gone, to be replaced by Sister Sandra, who is in her mid-fifties and one of our less jolly members of staff. She has grey hair, thin hips and even thinner lips. I made the mistake of shaking her hand once: not only does she have the grip of Lennox Lewis, but her skin is so rough and dry it could take the paint off a car. I'm not sure what she has done to them over the years but they are clearly not great pals with hand cream.

'Where have you been?' she asks.

'The lavatory,' I find myself lying. When is she going to realize that I am not fresh out of medical school? That I start specialist training next year? Just because I have the face of a twenty-year-old choirboy who's never seen a razor, it doesn't mean I am one.

'Right, well, the consultant has been looking for you,' she says rather tartly. 'In one.' She looks across at the cubicle.

I draw back the curtain, and I have to say I am shocked by what I see. Lying on the bed is a white-faced young man with filthy matted hair, stained teeth and sores on his face and arms with the largest blown-up backside I have ever seen. It is huge, swollen like a beach ball; the skin is so red it has gone maroon and purple in parts.

Ian looks at me, his eyes rounded and slightly panicked.

'Andrew here,' he begins, his voice sounding remarkably controlled bearing in mind the situation, 'is an intravenous drugs user.'

'OK.'

'It appears that the heroin he's been using has been cut with warfarin.'

'What? Why would anyone cut heroin with blood thinner?'

'Who the hell knows? Anyway, there appears to be a lot of the stuff in the smack because he's come up with an INR eighteen.'

'*Eighteen?*'

I'm now finding it hard to believe the man is still alive. Normally an INR – or international normalized ratio, which determines the clotting tendency of blood – is 1. If you are thinning the blood down after a clot you'd aim for 2 to 3. A 4 would be high. I would have thought that 18 would be fatal. But apparently not.

'So I gave him an injection for pain relief,' continues Ian.

'Inter-muscular?' I check, as the situation dawns on me.

'Yup,' says Ian.

'OK,' I nod. And the patient has obviously seriously bled into the muscle and, as he can't clot properly, his backside is still filling with blood. If left alone in this state, Andrew's nerves and blood vessels will collapse and he will die. 'And the plan is . . . ?'

'The plan is to pump the patient with Beriplex, slice open the buttock and bleed him.'

'Bleed him?'

'Bleed him.'

So this is exactly what we do. It's like something out of a Victorian horror movie. Ian pumps the coagulant into Andrew, then sticks his scalpel in his butt-cheek and slices open the skin, which is under so much pressure from the blood pouring into the muscle that it bursts apart like an overly ripe piece of fruit. Blood sprays out of the small incision. It is clearly a relief for Andrew, who moans slightly and rolls his eyes. He is, of course, high as a kite on heroin and morphine, which I imagine must be quite a potent mixture. I'm not sure he can feel a thing, actually, maybe just the pressure of blood in his buttock. Connie is standing by, armed with wads and wads of swabs to soak up the flow of blood, which keeps on gushing out. The colour is draining even more from Andrew's face. His lips have gone blue. He looks like he is about to faint.

'Jesus,' I say. 'That's a lot of blood.'

'We worked out he had about three litres in his backside,' says Ian, now applying pressure to the wound, forcing the remaining blood out.

Andrew is going to have the most monumental bruise on his arse tomorrow when he wakes up on the ward. I wonder how many other junkies in the area have taken this dirty heroin. I'm pretty sure Andrew won't be the only one to get a massive haematoma with that amount of warfarin cut with the smack. He's one of the lucky ones. This really is lethal stuff.

It takes another fifteen minutes or so of squeezing the lanced buttock to get all the blood out. Fortunately, after a while the coagulant starts to kick in and slow down the bleeding. Andrew flops back on to his trolley. He will be admitted on the ward in a while, where he can be monitored. He's lost a lot of blood and will be feeling quite lousy for the next twenty-four hours or so – quite apart from the fact that he'll be coming down soon as well, having lost half his heroin hit through his backside. Not that it will teach him a lesson. I'm pretty sure we'll see him back here again in a couple of weeks.

If you stay here long enough you begin to get to know the faces. There are patients who come in here whom Chris, Ian and the other consultants know if not entirely by name, then at least by faces and symptoms – the junkies, the alkies, the prostitutes. It is never a question of curing them; your job is to patch them up and send them on their way so they can carry on their abusive lives. When I first came here I remember complaining to Chris what a pain in the arse they were, how they were nothing but trouble, a pointless waste of time, talent and resources. He told me that they weren't trouble, they were a challenge. He also reminded me that they were victims of life, that what we should do is turn back the clock and see how it all started. We should try to understand rather than sit in judgement. Some people were born victims, there was no question of that. But some were also weaker than others. They were simply not able to cope with what life had thrown at them. Some had fallen to the bottom of the pile because they didn't have the discipline or the strength of character to keep standing, to keep fighting. They were just not capable of sorting themselves out. I have to say that Chris is a much nicer, kinder doctor than I am. After all this time I still find it hard sometimes not to show my irritation.

I say goodbye to Chris as he is leaving and go to the changing room to put on my fourth set of scrubs today. There, I greet Sanjay and Alex, two more consultants who will be on now for the whole night. Sanjay is in his late forties and has been a consultant in A&E for about five years; Alex, around ten years younger, has just been given the post.

'I've heard you've had quite a day of it,' says Sanjay.

Born and trained in Delhi, Sanjay always says that he dreamt of being a doctor in the UK. Although these days he is seriously thinking about returning to India to set up a hospital on the outskirts of the city.

'A resurrection, no less,' he smiles.

'Good news travels fast,' I say, searching through the pile of scrubs for a large top.

'Not such great news for the transplant team,' adds Alex.

From the home counties and Cambridge-educated, Alex is one of the brightest new recruits in the team. He is also a bit of a hit with the physio girls, the nurses, and indeed all the girls. He is married with a brand-new baby daughter, but that doesn't stop anyone from trying.

'No, but good news for our stats,' says Sanjay.

'We've actually had two deaths already today,' I say. 'And we are still waiting for the debrief.'

'Really?' says Alex. 'I think it'll be tomorrow morning now.'

'Anything else we should know about?' asks Sanjay.

'We haven't got many on tonight,' I say. 'And I'm on a double.'

'Yeah,' says Alex, 'I wondered what you were still doing here. Can't keep away?'

'Well, you know,' I shrug, finally finding a top.

'Good dancing last night,' smirks Alex as he walks out

of the room. 'I didn't have you down as an Abba man.'

'Oh, I missed that moment,' says Sanjay as he follows Alex out into the corridor.

I leave them to it and have a quick look through my stuff for my iPhone. I need to send Emma a quick text just to tell her that I am working right through tonight and not to expect me home. Fortunately my phone is still in my jeans pocket wrapped in a handkerchief, where I left it. I have three missed calls, all from her. She's left one irate message. My text is brief and to the point and devoid of apology. To be honest, I'm not sure how long this relationship is going to last.

I can feel myself flagging a bit. The image of the teenage boy pouring blood from every inch of his body flashes in front of my mind. I need a cup of coffee before I go back in there. Sometimes it is hard to take the pace.

Melissa, one of the more functional anaesthetists, is sitting on a chair in the common room, speed-eating a sandwich while finishing off a sudoku puzzle on her lap.

'All right?' she asks, wiping her nose on the back of her hand.

'I'm a bit tired,' I reply.

'You and me both,' she says. 'I've been in the longest bloody operation this afternoon with the world's slowest bloody paediatric surgeon trying to cut a carcinoma out of a twelve-year-old's liver.'

'Sounds nasty.'

'It was. But the surgeon – do you know him, Geoff Bank?'

'Yes.'

'He was so fucking slow that the patient twitched and he

asked me if the child had moved and I said, "No, it's natural bloody growth!"' She takes a huge bite of her sandwich. 'I am so hungry I could eat two bloody horses.'

'Geoff's a bit old now,' I say.

'Old!' she snorts. 'I'm amazed he can still get insured.'

'Perhaps he can't,' I say. 'That's why he's working for us.'

'And he left a swab behind,' she adds.

It transpires that Geoff had asked the nurses three times to count the swabs and they'd insisted he had taken them all out. It wasn't until the final count at the end that they'd realized their mistake. Swabs and equipment always get counted in and out of an operation to prevent just what happened this afternoon. Of course it's not a foolproof system. There are endless stories of the most extraordinary things being left behind in bodies after operations – swabs, needles, screws, bolts. The guys dealing with big cavities have to be especially careful. Earlier this month one of the surgeons left a ruler inside someone's stomach; it was only after the patient complained of stomach ache that anyone bothered to check. There are a lot of people in theatre for the big operations and each has their own sometimes quite small part to play, so you can see how things can get lost. It's hard to make sure everything is done properly when the person who is ultimately accountable for running the show often leaves before the end.

'Anyway, we got it in the end,' she says. 'We had to open the poor boy up again to fish it out. Added another half-hour to the operation.'

'No wonder you're so hungry.'

'Starving. You on all night tonight?'

'Doing the graveyard,' I say.

'I'm off at ten,' she says, looking at the clock. 'Not long now.'

I leave Melissa to her sudoku and her sandwich and once more launch myself at the coalface of the community.

'You took your time,' says Sandra.

'I couldn't find any scrubs,' I lie again. What is it about this woman that puts my back up so much?

I walk over to the computer and click on the next patient.

The waiting room is surprisingly clear when I walk in. There is a distinct smell of McDonald's in the air. Two blokes in the far corner are demolishing the remnants of a quarter-pounder meal. There's an old man asleep; I'm not sure if he's actually waiting to be treated or just using the plastic seating as a convenient resting place. A group of teenage girls are texting in a row right in front of me. None of them bothers to look up. A drunk in a suit catches my eye, then tries to keep his own open.

'Mr Hughes?' I ask, looking around the room. 'Mr Hughes?'

A middle-aged man with brown floppy hair raises himself gingerly off the seat. He walks very slowly towards me. Each step is clearly quite painful for him. He huffs and puffs in little tiny breaths, trying to control his pain.

'Mr Hughes?' I check.

'Yes,' he just about manages to say.

'Severe abdominal pain?' I hazard, a little puzzled.

'Yes, yes,' he replies, sounding a little annoyed.

'I am sorry to have kept you waiting,' I say as I lead him to the consulting area.

'Two hours twenty minutes,' he says.

'Sorry about that,' I say again – it's practically a reflex action these days. 'If you'd like to pop yourself up on the bed then I'll take a look at your stomach.'

Mr Hughes slips off his brown leather shoes and very slowly crawls up on to the bed and lies back down. There is much inhaling and exhaling and wincing. He is obviously in a lot of pain. He pulls his shirt up to reveal what appears to be a totally normal stomach. I stand above him and start pressing the abdomen, checking for any irregularities. Then I stop. I can feel something weird. He seems to be vibrating from the inside.

'I'm sorry, Mr Hughes,' I say, 'but you appear to be buzzing.'

'Yes,' he says. 'I can explain.'

9–10 p.m.

It seems that Mr Hughes was having an amusing and sexually inventive afternoon with his lover/secretary. They had booked into a hotel room, around the corner from the hospital, and got themselves some entertainment from Ann Summers, including a French maid's outfit, a large tub of lube and one purple dildo. The lover/secretary had put the maid's outfit on and covered Mr Hughes in lube before switching the dildo to super-vibrate and popping it up Mr Hughes's backside. He is then at a loss to explain quite how she let go of the dildo, or quite how it slipped so far inside, but suffice to say it did. According to the X-rays I have just got back, it has progressed rather a long way up the anal canal. Indeed, the particular alchemy of vibration and peristalsis means that the Bliss 8 Vibe is quite speedily making its way up beyond the sigmoid colon and into the large intestine.

'How long have you had the vibrator up there?' I ask.

'Four or five hours,' replies Mr Hughes, shifting

uncomfortably on the bed. 'We spent about an hour trying to get it out by ourselves but then Sally had to go home – to her husband.'

'Right. Should I call your wife?'

'No!' he says, immediately.

'But the thing is, you are going to be here for some time,' I say.

'Can't you just put some gloves on and pull it out?' he asks. I can hear the panic rising in his voice.

'I'm afraid it has gone a bit far for that.' I pause. 'We need to wait for it to run out of batteries, I think.'

'No, we can't,' he objects. 'We've used long-life ones. You know, like with the pink bunny that carries on drumming for ever?' He looks like he is about to weep as the awfulness of his situation dawns on him.

'You need an operation,' I say. 'We need to call in a specialist.'

He nods.

'A proctologist,' I add.

'A what?'

'A doctor who deals in the lower gut.'

He looks confused.

'They're called bums and tums doctors.'

'A man who just deals with arseholes?' he asks.

'Not just arseholes. Arseholes and other things.'

Mr Hughes flops back on to the bed. I swear I have never seen a man more miserable or depressed. A silly sexy afternoon with his secretary has resulted in him having to have an arse op, and probably a very serious discussion indeed with his wife. And hopefully he's one of the lucky ones at the end of it. There are plenty of patients who think it witty to shove something up their backsides only for them to damage themselves so badly they need a colostomy bag for ever after.

And it's not just vibrators that end up up there. Deodorant bottles, beer bottles, toilet brushes, carrots, leeks, turnips – any number of root vegetables, in fact, and anything with a handle. One of my favourites was a man who arrived in A&E with a carrot up his backside; when asked how he did it, he replied that he had fallen over while gardening. Clearly, in his eyes, gardening with no clothes on was more acceptable than buggery by vegetable. And sometimes the excuses are more interesting than the presentation. Another middle-aged man (it is always middle-aged men with things up their backsides, and they are more often than not straight; it seems gay men know what they are doing a little better) arrived with a tennis ball very firmly wedged up his bottom. Before the anaesthetic, the surgeon asked him how he did it, and the man explained that he went downstairs naked in the middle of the night to get something from the sitting room. He was standing by the fireplace, and when he bent down to pick up what he had forgotten, a tennis ball fell off the mantelpiece, bounced, and shot up his parted buttocks. No one believed him, of course. The surgeon then instructed the anaesthetist to ask him the same question as he came round after the anaesthetic. All of us tell the truth at that moment of complete vulnerability. The anaesthetist did as he was told, and the man came up with exactly the same answer!

It also seems that in a fit of passion, or indeed insanity, any hole will do. I remember spending one New Year's Eve pulling a balloon out of someone's bladder. I have no idea how it got up there, or why you would want to put a balloon up your penis, or how you could derive any sexual pleasure from it. I am also not sure if the idea was to inflate it afterwards. But I am pretty sure the bloke won't be doing it again. The whole thing proved to be very painful, and I think it was over a month before he was able to piss straight.

And it's not only men who go in for the insertion of foreign objects. Last year there was a student nurse who quite frankly should have known better. She was from Poland so maybe one's kicks are a little different there, but she came in with a shattered light bulb up her fanny. Apparently she had been warming it up by turning the light on, then she'd taken the warm bulb out and had been using it to pleasure herself when the thing broke. Needless to say it was all a bit of a mess. I also remember fishing around in a woman's vagina for a squash ball one tricky afternoon. I tell you, after half an hour of look- ing, it made you realize why tampons have strings. When I finally got it out, all anyone in A&E wanted to know was what speed the ball was. For the record, it was a blue spot, which I think is the fastest you can get.

'You're in luck,' says Ian, poking his head around the curtain. 'I've managed to get Mr Armstrong out of a dinner round the corner. He's going to be here in about twenty minutes.'

'Mr Armstrong?' asks Mr Hughes.

'One of the best proctologists in the country,' I tell him. 'You are honoured.'

'You say that,' he replies, wincing slightly. He looks completely defeated and utterly mortified.

I decide to give him some space – the last thing Mr Hughes needs is someone constantly checking up on his humiliation. He has been alone for all of two seconds when Melissa comes up the corridor looking a lot jollier since her tuna sandwich, closely followed by Ben.

'Your patient,' she says. 'Vibrator up the rectum?' She checks on her list. 'Do you know if he has eaten anything?'

'I didn't ask, I'm afraid.'

'Alcohol?'

'Not that I can smell.'

'No one puts a purple rubber cock up their arse if they're sober,' says Ben.

'Oh I don't know,' says Melissa, and disappears behind the curtain.

'She's got to be a goer,' says Ben, tapping the side of his nose.

'I haven't had much to do with her, I'm afraid.'

'Shame,' says Ben. 'She's got lovely tits.'

'Really?'

'You have really got to be more observant,' he says. 'I hear we have the King of Bums coming in,' he continues. 'We're probably tearing him away from an Upper Gut Society dinner.'

'Or a Lower Gut Society dinner,' I add.

'Or a Vascular Society do, or an Association of Surgeons buffet,' he laughs.

'I bet none of that lot have attended a buffet in twenty years,' I add.

Right at the top of the consultant food chain, the air gets very rarefied. The lunches get longer, the operations get shorter, the offices are obviously larger and the cars get very fat indeed. Mr Armstrong is hugely in demand. He is invited all over the world to chat to other splendid surgeons who are also in demand, and he gets paid for it. His earnings are touching, if not over, the million-pound mark. His list of private clients is global. He deals in international arseholes and is remunerated accordingly. He has a Harley Street practice, and if he can keep getting insured he'll carry on with that until way after he has finished keeping his hand in with the NHS.

'It's a weird specialism, dealing entirely with backsides,' I observe. 'I wonder if he finds it hard to remember his patients' faces.'

'I don't know,' says Ben. 'I think the more you specialize in this business, the more interesting it becomes. I was at a Christmas party last year and I met a doctor who specializes in bum enlargements. He spends twenty-eight days a year in Trinidad and Tobago putting silicone pads into patients' butt cheeks and the rest of the year he plays golf. Occasionally he is flown somewhere to speak; sometimes he might come in and fill some cancerous-tumour cavity on the NHS just to make himself feel a little better, and remind himself he is not a total charlatan. What a perfect life.' He looks around the strip-lit hall we are both standing in which stinks of piss, booze and disinfectant. 'But sadly no one told me at medical school that you could specialize in arse enlargements. They say variety is the spice of life, but not in the medical world. If you choose variety, you end up here. ' We both look around. 'The truth is, the more specialized you are, the more fantastic your life is. If you do eyelids, for example, you end up flying to LA to do half of Hollywood. You'd think it would be dull doing one thing, but intrinsically everything is interesting.'

'What would you like to do?'

'I quite fancy being an orthopaedic surgeon.'

'Really?' I'd always thought that one of the more dull specialisms, looking after fractures, broken ankles and twisted knees.

'Yeah, then I could have a private practice specializing in sports injuries and operate on the Chelsea football team.'

'In Harley Street?'

'That's overrated,' he says.

Actually, he's right about that. Harley Street is a bit over-rated these days. Although it's getting better than it was. Its reputation has become tarnished a little over the years, mainly due to the high rents and the widespread practice of sub-letting. A large proportion of Harley Street properties are owned by the Howard De Walden Estate, which is extremely careful who it rents to, as are the Crown Estates that also own swathes of the area. However, this did not preclude doctors renting properties and then sub-letting them to other doctors, which led to the practice of hot-desking or hot-officing. So a doctor could say he has a Harley Street address and consultation suite when in fact he only uses it on a Thursday afternoon between three and six p.m. The powers-that-be have recently woken up to this and are trying to clamp down on it, but when the rents are £6,000 a month for two small treatment rooms, you can kind of see why it happens. For the same amount of money you can have ten rooms on Wimpole Street. But it just doesn't have the same cachet.

Weirdly, where you are on Harley Street dictates how much your rent is. The lower the number, the more it costs. Number 1 Harley Street is the most expensive address in the street, whereas 150 will be at least 30 per cent less expensive to rent.

'I wouldn't say it's overrated,' says Sanjay, joining in. 'It has a worldwide reputation. I have a friend who does plastic surgery on the street and he says he can't move anywhere else. For Arabic patients from the Middle East, Great Britain means three things: Harrods, Knightsbridge, for shopping; Edgware Road for the hubble-bubble; and Harley Street for medicine. Oh, and Regent's Park is the countryside.' He laughs. 'It's true. If you tell them to take their bloods to Wimpole Street they say it is too far. If you ask them to come to Devonshire Place, they get completely lost.'

'You would have thought all those Botox places would've taken a kicking in the recession,' I say.

'You're kidding, right?' says Ben. 'Lots of the small country clinics are going bankrupt, but all the good places like my mate's place are packed. Their billions may have become millions, but women for whom Botox and fillers are the norm don't feel dressed without it. It's like going to the hairdresser's for them. Also, famously, lipstick sales go up in a recession: you may not be able to afford the shoes and the dress but you are sure as hell going to keep your lips pillow perfect.'

'I always think they look disgusting, those big fat lips, like you've been in a fight with your orthodontist,' I say.

'I know,' agrees Sanjay. 'But the big lips are very popular with the Arabic women. They're used to wearing very heavy make-up. Like us in Delhi, they like their movie stars with big features, so they like the big lips and the big cheekbones.'

'And the Russians are hilarious,' adds Ben. 'They are so designer-obsessed that they ask for their fillers by brand, so they insist on Sculptra instead of another derma-filler.'

'And the Brits like boob-job tits,' says Sanjay. 'Ones that actually look fake. We can do much better tit jobs these days, but still you lot want them hard and with a runway in the middle like a WAG. They are a status symbol, not a thing of beauty!'

Melissa comes out from behind the curtain, and I am afraid to say we all stand and stare at her breasts. Ben does so because he knows they are great, I do because I'm checking out Ben's recommendation, and Sanjay does so because he's talking about British boobs. We all fix our gaze and tacitly agree they are rather good.

'All right?' she says, staring at the three of us staring at her. She is a little confused.

'Yes, very good,' I say. 'You?'

'Very good. Two glasses of champagne and five chocolate-coated strawberries since breakfast,' she says. 'I think I can work with that.'

'Oh yes, right,' I say, suddenly realizing what she is talking about. 'I think I'd better go and see if Mr Armstrong has arrived yet.'

'Do you need to?' she asks.

'Yup,' I say. Anything to get out of this situation.

I arrive outside the front of the hospital to see a black Ferrari sports car pull up on the yellow zigzags. Extremely loud classical music is pouring out of the open window. The engine stops, as does the music, and a lean, neat, handsome white-haired gent nips out the opposite side of the car. I know he must be knocking sixty, or indeed over it, but he looks fit enough to beat a twenty-year-old in a triathlon. He locks the car with a swift bleep and throws an expensive-looking dinner jacket over his shoulder. He has undone the dickie bow, and he's sporting a pair of highly polished shoes. He also has one of those leathered, weathered deep tans that only comes after many winter top-ups on a Florida golf course.

'Mr Armstrong?' I say.

'It's all right here, is it, the car,' he states rather than asks.

'Absolutely,' I agree.

'Don't you just love Haydn?' he asks in a manner that demands you agree. So I do, even if I can't name a single piece of his music. 'Excellent,' he says, patting me on the back. 'Very important to have some good music while you operate.'

'I do hope we haven't dragged you away from something important,' I say.

'Oh, just another one of those dinners where you eat indeterminate fowl in an indeterminate sauce and show off how many papers you've written. I was sitting next to the wife of the surgeon who had written the haemorrhoid chapter in some new compendium. It was riveting.' He roars with laughter. It's loud and raucous, the sort to make small babies cry. 'Anyway, fill me in on our dear patient.'

We walk and talk and I explain to Mr Armstrong exactly how far up the colon the purple vibrator has managed to work itself.

'What is it with heterosexual men and their bottoms?' he

asks loudly as he walks up the stairs. 'Last week, at another hospital that I cover, I had a company director who had a carrot up his rear, inside a French letter. I did think about asking him how it got up there but I just couldn't be bothered to listen to a poorly worked-through story.'

'I'm sure it gets rather tiresome after a while,' I say.

'No,' he says. 'There are certain little things that are sent by the Lord to amuse you. I took a pepper pot out of another backside a few years back, and down one side it said "Welcome to Margate". That tickled me for weeks. I have had a small statuette of Napoleon, a Brighton pier, a Blackpool Tower a few times. And a couple of sticks of rock.'

'I sense a seaside theme,' I say.

He rocks with laughter and slaps me on the back again.

'Of course I don't just remove foreign objects from the rectum,' he says.

The poor bloke is one of the leading specialists in bowel cancer and reconstructs a bowel so brilliantly that the majority of his patients don't leave wearing a bag. He is extremely talented, and to be honest I am a little embarrassed at his being here.

'I tell you one thing about my profession over the other more glamorous surgeries.' He smiles, then lowers his voice. 'They are always very grateful. One of the sad things is that everyone leaves their diagnosis much later than most other things due to embarrassment. They are prepared to suffer symptoms they wouldn't accept anywhere else out of mortification. So by the time they get to me, they are often quite desperate.'

Before he meets another grateful customer, I take him to one side to show him the X-rays. He switches on the light box opposite the computer and nearly the whole department comes to take a look. The dildo is huge and there for all to see, including the outline of the two long-life batteries. A few people giggle at the sight, most people wince, and there are a couple of sharp intakes of breath.

'That is quite far up,' he agrees. 'I'm not sure that is quite the result he intended when he popped it in this afternoon.'

'Do you think we should leave it in until the batteries run out?' I ask.

'Not unless we want to leave him with permanent damage,' he replies. 'They are quite determined, these things. Once they get going it's hard to stop them. It's travelled far enough already.'

'Then it might get nasty,' I say, staring at the bizarre X-ray. Why would you want to do that to yourself?

'That's not nasty,' insists Mr Armstrong. 'One of the worst things I've seen is a man who used to enjoy lowering himself on to the shaft end of a feather duster using a stepladder. Until one fine day the stepladder slipped and the broom ended up in his neck. His guts were transfixed. He had speared himself with a feather duster.'

A hush goes over the small gathering by the X-ray light box. A few stare open-mouthed at Mr Armstrong. He continues to look at the plates, somewhat oblivious to the fallout from his story.

'Did he live?' a nurse asks finally.

'Don't be ridiculous,' barks Mr Armstrong. 'DOA. Let's go and talk to our Mr Hughes, shall we?'

10–11 p.m.

I leave Mr Armstrong to discuss the pros and cons and possible outcomes of the bum op with Mr Hughes. He is no longer my patient, though I will of course come and check him over after he has come out of theatre. I think I might use this quick opportunity to go, via the changing room, and grab an over-priced sandwich from downstairs. The main canteen is closed now, which I always find a little annoying as this place is open twenty-four hours a day. Apparently there isn't much call for toad in the hole and chicken curry at three a.m., but I beg to disagree. So we have to make do with the small selection of sandwiches available at the shitty kiosk on the right as you come into the hospital. There is a fridge to the left of the till that boasts month-old Ginsters pies on one shelf and a few cheese and tomato sandwiches on the shelf below. Chilled within an inch of their lives, they are usually wet and soggy by this time of day as they near the end of, or indeed pass, their shelf life. They occasionally have a wrap, with something tandoori'd inside, but I refuse to eat a wrap. It's like chewing a dank newspaper and so goddamn depressing.

On the ground floor, the place is empty and the lights have been turned down low. It's almost like the hospital pretends to be closed, deterring as many 'customers' as it can. There are two blokes sitting at the front desk, both reading free-sheets with their feet up on the desk. A few flickering TV screens in front of them show various corridors, doorways and car parks; neither of them is paying much attention.

'Evening,' I say.

Neither of them bothers to look up, let alone reply.

On the far side of the entrance hall, a cleaner polishes the lino floor. He is wearing earphones, the music turned up loud against the polisher's low hum. He looks up at me, but his face does not react in the slightest. I am invisible to him. He checks the clock on the wall above my head before turning his back and carrying on.

In the shop, which the hospital sub-lets to claw back a tiny bit of income, the assistant is asleep. He is sitting on one of those wheelie footstools, leaning against a pile of old newspapers. The shop actually closes at ten p.m. but since he has failed to shut up properly I am hoping he might serve me.

I grab a soft white sandwich from the fridge. I don't even care what's inside it. 'Evening,' I say. 'Can I just have this?'

The man rubs his eyes. 'Three pounds,' he says.

'Three?' It's almost worth leaving the building and popping to the nearby twenty-four-hour garage. Such a rip-off.

'Three,' he repeats, sticking his dry, cracked hand out for good measure.

I feel a surge of irritation. If I weren't so hungry and pushed for time, I might just chuck the soggy thing back in his face. I put down the three coins I pulled from my jeans pocket a few minutes ago and tear open the plastic packet. It's tuna and cucumber – at least that's what it vaguely tastes like. I'm not entirely sure. The textures are wrong, and I'm sure that if I looked at the ingredients carefully I'd see that some sort of substitute has been used for the crucial elements. But right now I don't care and I have finished the thing before the lift arrives to take me back up to the first floor.

Once inside A&E I am presented with my first pisshead of the night. According to Sandra, who fills me in as I burp into the back of my hand, he was found in a car park by the police, out cold, next to what they presume is his car. He is too drunk to give his name, he can barely stand, and it took two nurses to 'walk' him into the cubicle. The shocking thing is, he is wearing a shirt and tie and the label inside his suit says Paul Smith. So the bloke must have a bit of money. Where are his mates? Where are his work colleagues? Why didn't someone see he got home? How does someone let themselves get so drunk that they pass out in a car park next to their own car? And he does stink of alcohol – the sweet heady smell of too much wine. I have to say, over the years that I have been doing this job, I have grown to hate that smell. I know it's hypocritical because I was drunk last night too. But this smell combined with the disinfectant and the strip lights . . . it's just such an unpalatable combination.

215

To be honest, alcohol is the bane of our lives in this place. Alcohol-related admissions have doubled since 2006, accounting for over eight hundred thousand of the cases we have to deal with, and costing the NHS more than £2.7 billion a year. Quite apart from the fact that it is completely self-inflicted, it's the bad behaviour, the abuse, the fights, the insults, the shouting, the spitting, the vomiting and the pissing that goes with the alcohol that makes it so annoying.

The police are also quite naughty: they bring a passed-out drunk to A&E simply because they don't know what to do with them. The police cells are full, and they can't be bothered to charge them for being drunk and disorderly. Short of driving them home like a very reliable cab service, they have no option but to bring them here. We are then, of course, obliged to check them over for head injuries and see if they have damaged themselves in some way before administering 'fluids'.

There are two schools of thought about fluids. The first is, give them as many fluids as possible in order to dilute the alcohol, sober them up and get them on their way so that we can have the bed back as we are not running an alternative B&B service. The second is, don't give them too many fluids as they will only end up pissing themselves and then we'll have something else to clear up. There is of course a third view: give them as many fluids as you can in order that they do actually piss themselves and therefore humiliate themselves into never, ever getting so completely drunk again. Sadly, the one flaw in this, apart from having to clear up a whole load of urine, is that some people don't have a very sensitive bladder reflex when drunk, so instead of peeing automatically when the bladder is full they end up rupturing their bladders, which is a whole new ball game.

This dignified end to a night, resulting in major surgery and someone stitching together your exploded nether regions, used to be an entirely male preserve and completely unheard of in women. But now they are catching up. The number of women drinking regularly currently stands at 86 per cent, which is almost the same as blokes, of whom 91 per cent are regular boozers. So it's only a matter of time before we have as many female bladder accidents as male.

The orderlies have wheeled Mr Hughes off for his bum op and taken both Gabriella and Andrew up into the ward to recover from their ordeals, thankfully freeing up some space; which is fortunate because my drunken suit suddenly jerks himself up off the bed and sprays half the section in vomit.

'Oh Jesus Christ!' says Stacy as she looks down at her blue tunic covered in yellow bile, diced carrots and half-digested pizza. 'I've only just put this on!'

I have to say I feel exactly the same. I'm now beginning to forget how many times I've changed today. Thank God he missed my shoes. I've never been one for putting on the bag feet, and there's nothing worse than squelching about in puke for the rest of your shift.

Sandra is straight out of the office, her thin face now looking even more pinched and grim. She rustles up cleaners and mops from nowhere, while Stacy and I walk off to change.

'And so it begins,' she says to me, wrinkling her small nose.

'I know,' I sympathize. 'And I thought tonight might be quiet.'

'You *hoped* it might.' She smiles. 'This is me,' she says, going into the ladies' changing room.

Five minutes later there's a knock on the door of the blokes' changing room and Stacy walks straight in before I have a chance to say anything.

'Are you ready yet, doctor?' she asks, smiling as she catches me in my scrubs trousers looking, yet again, through the pile for a top my size.

'Um, not quite there, actually,' I say, feeling my cheeks redden.

She deals with and looks at naked people all the time; why am I embarrassed for her to see me without my top on?

'Do you want a hand?' she asks, coming closer. 'What are you? A large or an' – she licks her lips lightly – 'extra large?'

'Just a large,' I say, trying not to catch her eye.

The thing is, Stacy is quite sexy. She is tall and slim, with dark bobbed hair and a whiff of a Scottish accent. I just never expected her ever to come on to me. I know she's been around the department a bit but she has never shown any interest in me before. I silently thank the Lord for the 'Black Wednesday effect' . . . and then, rather annoyingly, an image of Emma pops into my head.

'Here you go,' she says, flapping out a top and coming even closer. 'This is your size.'

''Ello, 'ello, what's going on in here?' comes a voice.

Another doctor, Mark, marches straight in through the door. Stacy and I leap apart.

'Call me old-fashioned, but I was under the impression this was a gents' changing area for changing gents.'

'I was just helping,' says Stacy, giving me a wink as she walks out.

'Evening, Dr Death,' I say. 'I didn't know we had the pleasure of you tonight.'

'Last night only,' he grins.

Mark is called Dr Death because, surprisingly enough, he killed someone. The person died at the end of his needle after he drew up a massive dose of potassium instead of painkiller, which stopped the patient's heart. He was a junior at the time, a student fresh out of medical school; it wasn't actually on Black Wednesday but he had only just started. The hospital didn't so much cover it up as suck it up. He was never investigated. He was never suspended. They just said 'Don't do it again' and he carried on. I have to say that even now, some four years later, I'm not that keen on having him on the shift with me. Some people think he's bad luck to have around; I just think he's not so much incompetent as a little bit crap. And he's a bit of a dickhead, too. The sort of person who gives you the two-fingered pistol-shoot greeting across the canteen. Anyway, I tend to try and give him a wide berth.

'You on tonight, then?' I ask, pulling my scrubs top over my chest.

'Yup,' he says. 'Ten till six, that's me.' He looks me up and down. 'They really are serving up the dregs tonight.'

I leave the murdering idiot to put his scrubs on and go back out to A&E to check on my drunk. There's only a residual smell of vomit in the area, mixed with a more potent smell of alcohol and disinfectant – the usual evening aroma sported by the department. The bloke is passed out, snoring on the bed, with an IV of fluids in his arm. The vomiting has clearly done him some good as he looks a little less red and sweaty and on the verge of a heart attack. Although he looks a little better, he still has to sleep off his drinking binge, and as we won't admit him to the hospital, he is going to lie there and block a cubicle because there is nowhere else to put him.

'Hi there,' says Sanjay, poking his head around the curtain. 'If you're not busy I'd like you to come and scrub in with my patient.'

'I'm not sure I can,' I say. 'What's the problem?'

'A bleed behind a breast augmentation. I've got to take the bag out, stop the bleed and check to see if the bags themselves are punctured. She says they are saline bags but it's been done on the cheap, so we need to make sure she's not leaking silicone into her system.'

'OK,' I say. 'Where did she have it done?'

He names a clinic I've never heard of, but then there's no change there. Half these clinics come and go all the time; they run out of money and close, they get a poor rep and close. Some 66 per cent of them are not properly equipped and only 22 per cent of them have a resus team on all the time. We are endlessly clearing up after botched bloody plastic jobs.

They are almost as bad as the Independent Sector Treatment Centres, which are the bugbear of Chris Williams. Set up over five years ago, these private clinics, paid for by the NHS, are where so-called bulk operations are performed. The doctors who work there are not vetted in the way we are and are supposedly much less experienced. They also don't have the same aftercare system we do. Chris is always complaining about having to sort things out after some doctor has flown over on Ryanair, rattled off some botch job and pissed off again. He says the worst thing about many of these doctors is that they don't actually kill their patients, they maim them, leaving us with hours of corrective surgery to clean up their mess. We've had cases of hysterectomies without consent; of knee and hip ops done so badly we've had to replace the whole joint. One terrible statistic states that if you have a hip op at an ISTC you are twenty times more likely to have to have it repaired on the NHS.

Not that we are beyond reproach ourselves of course. We have quacks like Dr Death still walking, talking and working among us. Only six months ago we had a bit of a problem with the operating theatres. Patients kept on getting post-operative infections so the whole place was cleaned and disinfected and sterilized over and over again, and still it kept on happening. Eventually they managed to get the resident microbiologist to grow some of the bacteria, and to everyone's amazement it was faecal. After much toing and froing and asking around, the outbreak was whittled down to one surgical registrar who had terrible piles and was itching his arse during operations.

Sanjay disappears off to find someone else to assist him when Melissa comes up to inform me that Mr Hughes has come through OK and is coming round in the recovery room at the end of the corridor. When I walk in I am met with the usual sight of about six gently moaning bodies lying flat out on trolleys. I am always struck by how much this place, devoid of the mumbling and the beeping machines, reminds me of the morgue. I think it's the thin yellow curtains that hang between each body, or the fact that they're all laid out. Either way, it always freaks me out a bit.

Mr Hughes is lying next to an intubated woman with an oxygen mask over her face; she is motionless and looks extremely uncomfortable. Mr Hughes is turned on his side. I imagine he'll be sleeping in this position for some time to come. I don't think the operation was particularly complicated, but it must have been rather painful. Mr Hughes will be kept in, certainly overnight and possibly for another twenty-four hours after that. He certainly won't be allowed to leave until he has passed a normal stool. I look over his charts. His stats are all fine; he seems to be well.

'How are you, Mr Hughes?' I ask.

'Fine,' he says, sounding very sorry for himself.

'A little uncomfortable?' I ask.

'Mmm.'

'Good, well then, you'll be going on a ward soon,' I say. 'We'll keep you down here for half an hour or so just to make sure everything's OK, then we'll move you.'

'Mmm,' he says again.

'OK,' I say. 'Is there anything else?'

'Yes,' he says, suddenly and rather sharply. 'Can you get rid of the thing on the end of my bed?'

I look at the foot of his bed and in a glass jar, the sort of thing we use to store gallstones or tumours that patients want to keep, is the vibrator. Mr Armstrong is either being a little bit wicked, or he genuinely thinks that Mr Hughes might want to take the big purple cock home with him as a souvenir. My money's on wicked.

'If you're sure?' I ask, picking up the vibrator-in-a-jar.

'Completely,' he says, curling himself up into a tight ball.

I walk back down the corridor holding the glass jar. I'm not quite sure what to do with it. I suppose technically it's surgical waste and should be incinerated, along with the sharps, swabs and other unpleasant detritus.

'Oh, what's that?' asks Ben as he bumps into me.

I hold it up for closer inspection.

'Is that going into the girls' changing room? You should put a sticker on it: "In case of emergency, break glass".' He laughs. 'I'm sure they'd find it useful.'

'I think technically I should throw it away.'

We both inspect it a little more closely.

'It's not that clean,' I add, recoiling slightly.

'No,' he agrees, his nose curling. 'Definitely one for the bin.'

I am just disposing of the vibrator in a yellow clinical waste bucket in the cubicle next to my drunk when Mark sticks a rather sweaty-looking face around the curtain.

'Fuck, man! You've got to help me,' he says, staring down at his bloody rubber-clad hands. 'I've got some Saudi monoglot next door who's got a nose that just won't bloody stop bleeding.'

I obviously look at him with a puzzled expression.

'Help me! He's dying!'

I follow him through the curtain to find an elderly Arabic gentleman lying on the bed dressed in flowing white robes, with blood pouring out of his nose. It is rare to die of a nose-bleed. You have to lose a lot of blood out of a relatively small exit. It's not like being stabbed. There really has to be a substantial flow. But this man looks well on the way. His face is drained of colour and he looks weak and feeble, not long for this world.

'How long has he been like this?' I hiss.

'I don't fucking know,' says Mark, wringing his hands slightly. The man is panicking. 'I don't know how to stop it either. I mean, every single bit of cotton I've stuffed up there is just soaking it up. We've run out. Connie's gone to get more.'

'Here you are!' says Connie, arriving all red-faced and equally panicked.

'I mean, he's going to be dead in ten minutes if someone doesn't fucking do something fast,' announces Mark. His thinning blond hair is stuck to his head. 'Is Ian still here? He'd know what to do.'

'I can actually speak English you know,' comes a voice.

Mark, Connie and I all stare at the patient.

'Oh,' says Mark.

'Oh,' I repeat. 'I was told that you didn't.'

'He presumed,' continues the patient. 'I am an English teacher, actually. And this has happened to me many times before. What you need to do is this . . .'

I leave a completely mortified Mark to take instructions from his patient on how to stem the rampant blood flow and go next door to check on my drunk. I peel back the curtains and take a peek. I sigh. The man is fast asleep, his mouth is wide open, he's snoring like a trucker, and he has wet his trousers.

224

11 p.m.–12 a.m.

Stacy and I debate whether to leave my drunk, Richard, in his clothes. Stacy has been through his jacket pockets and worked out that he doesn't live that far from the hospital.

'I think I might go through his phone and call someone to come and get him,' she says, holding his mobile. 'I mean, he really is cluttering up the place, vomiting and urinating everywhere.'

'Have a go,' I agree. 'And as soon as he can sit up, get rid of him to the CDU.'

I'm not sure how many patients are sitting in the clinical decision unit at the moment, but I'm sure Ian, Alex and Sanjay will have offloaded a few by now. I walk through the A&E waiting room to check.

The CDU is even more grubby than the A&E waiting room, mainly because it's completely devoid of frills. There is no TV, no table full of jaded, dog-eared magazines and crumpled free-sheets, no water-cooler, in fact nothing but six rows of red plastic chairs and a slowly atrophying spider plant. Asleep in one corner is a drunk who I think Ian bagged, tagged and dispatched almost as soon as the man could sit up without slumping sideways. There's a man with a bandaged arm who also looks like he's sleeping off the effects of a liquid lunch, tea and dinner. There's also a granny who is pacing around, undoubtedly crazy with a kidney infection. The corridors of this hospital are always full of old ladies who have made themselves ill by forgetting to drink enough water. They wander around, waiting to be seen, waiting for someone to take any notice, or even sometimes, if they are lucky, waiting for the antibiotics to kick in. This granny is rather frail and extremely little. She must be all of five foot and she looks like she's knocking on the door of eighty.

'All right, dear?' I ask, bending down to her height.

'Is that you?' She stares at me. 'Graham? Is that you?'

'Hello there,' I say. 'I am not Graham. Has anyone seen you in the hospital?' I gently take her hand and look her over. She has a couple of plasters on her arms, which means she must have had some IV antibiotics. 'Who treated you?'

She looks blank.

'The name of your doctor?'

She looks like she's trying to think. Her lined grey forehead frowns. 'Graham,' she suggests.

'I think I'll go and take a look,' I say. 'You stay there.'

'Here,' she says.

Poor woman, I think as I walk back towards the department, she really doesn't know if it's Tuesday night or breakfast time. She's so elderly and vulnerable I'm not sure she should really be left anywhere on her own, least of all a grotty CDU with little or no supervision.

The waiting room is looking surprisingly unpacked, I think as I come through the doors. It's increasingly airless and the smell of fast food is slowly being trounced by beer, cheap wine and whisky.

'Hello there, handsome!' comes a familiar voice.

I turn round to see Emma standing in the doorway with her mate Jilly.

'Hi there!' Jilly waves.

'Muhammad couldn't get out to play with the mountain, so the mountain has come to see you!' declares Emma as she weaves her way towards me and kisses me on the cheek.

The kiss is wet, and she stinks of booze. I feel my stomach tighten slightly; my mouth goes dry as it dawns on me: she smells like a patient. There is something about her being here, slightly drunk, under the cold light of the neon strips, that makes me feel nauseous. I'm not annoyed that she's here. If she were sober, I'd be pleased to see her. But the smell and the state of her make me want to dump her right here and now. It's irrational, I know, but I can't help it.

She runs her hands over my cheeks and squeezes one of them, like I'm two years old. It makes my skin crawl.

'Don't you look all sweet in your jumpsuit,' she giggles.

'He looks sexy,' Jilly joins in. 'Just like George Clooney!'

'Help me, doctor!' says Emma, clutching her right breast. 'I think I might have a heart problem!'

'It's the other side,' I say.

227

'Of course it is!' She bursts out laughing.

'God, you'd make a shit nurse!' yelps Jilly.

Half the waiting room have stopped whatever fascinating thing they were doing and are watching the show.

'But I'd look great in a uniform,' Emma says, pouting and pulling her shirt low at the front and squashing her breasts together. She messes up her hair, licks her lips and tries to look sexy. She just ends up looking more drunk.

I have to say I am now beginning to fight feelings of deep revulsion. There is nothing I'd like more in the world right now than for her and her pissed-up pal to fuck off.

Working here really affects your personal life in ways you could not possibly imagine. Quite apart from the long hours, the high stress, and the matter-of-fact attitude you have to things like cannulating yourself and popping extremely strong cocktails of drugs to make you sleep, keep awake or just plain feel a little bit better, we also become inured to a lot of things. After you have seen life and death at its most raw, visceral and gruesome, you become cauterized, so much so that it is often quite hard to get emotional about anything. Bizarrely, we are part of society, at its front line most of the time, yet we are also isolated from the rest of the world. The intensity of our shift means that something could happen on the outside and we would not know anything about it until some six or eight hours later. Some mates of mine only found out about 9/11 four hours after the event, and that was only because A&E was suddenly empty: everyone had gone home to watch the telly.

All this impacts in obvious ways on our personal lives, but sometimes in ways you might never think of. Plenty of surgeons I know, in fact most of them, have a dislike of the naked human body. We don't find it sexy or alluring. I think it's because we associate it with work, or possibly problems. All I know is this: if you want to turn on a surgeon, flash some flesh, show a shoulder or some ankle, but keep your clothes on. Most of us like a woman in underwear. I think we have spent so long trying to desexualize the bodies we operate on that a prostrate naked form is no longer attractive. And woe betide anyone who is going out with or is married to a gynaecologist. Imagine what looking at fannies all day does to you. And as Sanjay pointed out a few weeks ago when we were discussing this very thing, they are not necessarily fannies in good condition either, they have cysts, abscesses, fibroids or some such hideous complication. Eventually it does start to get in the way of your sex life.

Anyway, my pet hate, when I have not been drinking myself, is the stench of alcohol. If I had been out and about with Emma my reaction to her flirting and pouting in front of me would have been different. But I have been working now for sixteen hours. I've seen two people die, and witnessed a resurrection. I have been covered in blood three times and puked on once. So you can imagine how jolly and well developed my sense of humour is right now. Quite apart from the fact that the patients are beginning to stare. I need to command respect from these people. I need them to think I'm infallible, that not only is my opinion valid, it should not be questioned.

'What do you think, doctor? Shall I take your blood pressure?'

Emma is smirking at me. Her eyeliner is smudged down her cheeks; her lipstick is bleeding into the tiny lines around her mouth. And she smells like a pub.

'How much have you had to drink?' I ask, fighting the waves of irritation that are coming thick and fast.

'Just a couple,' she says, wobbling slightly on her feet.

'Of bottles!' shrieks Jilly, falling backwards into a bin. 'Oops!' She laughs. 'I didn't see that there!'

'Can you just go,' I say, as quietly and firmly as I can.

'Go?' asks Emma. 'But we've just got here. We wanted you to show us around. Maybe have a look in the operating theatre.'

'Steal some drugs!' hoots Jilly, getting out of the bin.

They now have the attention of everyone in the waiting room – everyone who's still awake, that is.

'Can you please leave,' I say again, putting my hands on their shoulders, trying gently to usher them towards the double doors.

'There's no need to push me,' declares Emma, beginning to get annoyed that her late-night visit has not been received with open arms.

'I'm not.'

'You are!'

My heart sinks. Now she's going to get pissed off. Drunk and pissed off.

'Everyone's looking,' I say, still trying to corral them towards the door.

'Well let them!' laughs Jilly. 'What are you lot staring at?'

'Come on, please,' I say. I am prepared to beg.

'Get your hands off me,' says Emma. Her voice is raised. She is going to start shouting any minute.

'You heard the girl, doctor!' shouts Jilly, sticking up for her friend.

'I'm not touching you,' I say, putting my hands in the air, just wishing the whole thing would end – or had never started in the first place.

'Yes, you are!' yells Jilly.

'I'm not. Just please leave, the pair of you.'

They weave their way through the double doors, Emma looking extremely annoyed and tugging at her short skirt. She staggers slightly in her wedges and goes over on one ankle.

'You OK?' I ask after her.

'Fine,' she says, trying to walk like she's completely sober.

'I'm sorry,' I say as the doors close behind them. 'I'm working.'

'Fuck you!' she says, turning around. She walks off backwards while giving me the finger.

'Oops,' says Ben, appearing right next to me. 'That went well. Girlfriend?'

'Yes.'

'Not for much longer,' he says, sucking the back of his teeth, like a builder who's discovered rising damp.

'And I've only just got her,' I say.

'I wouldn't worry,' he says, patting me on the back, 'a good-looking bloke like you. I'm sure you could have your pick of the city's young ladies. And if not,' he smirks, 'there are always the nurses.'

It's weird watching Emma walk away. I'm not really sure

what she wanted me to do. Bring her into A&E to have a good gawp at some ill people? Show her where we put the corpses and have a fuck on the operating table? People have been known to shag in the operating theatre. It's nice and quiet, and you can close the door. But it's not my scene, I have to say. The bed's a bit narrow and I'm not that keen on the overhead lighting. Anyway, I'm sorry I disappointed her, but I wouldn't turn up at her office drunk, wanting a tour and a fumble in the filing cabinet in the middle of the day. Maybe it's because A&E is open to the public that she feels she has the right to just pop in whenever – much like everyone else, I suppose. We are paid for by the public, therefore we are public property. But I'm afraid it doesn't quite work like that.

'Hi, sorry,' says a very sweet-looking nurse who looks about twelve. 'You haven't seen a patient walk this way, have you?'

'A patient?' both Ben and I ask. Well, she is one of those nice-looking people you want to help.

'Yes,' she replies, her red-rimmed eyes darting up and down the corridor. 'She's, um, one of the prostitutes on the Hepworth Ward.'

Hepworth is one of the more notorious wards in the hospital. It's where we put all the intravenous drug users. We are in a difficult catchment area in the city, where there's quite a high number of heroin addicts. They are invariably homeless or prostitutes and are prone to a habit called skin-popping, a sort of last-resort form of injecting after all your veins have given up the ghost. The addict will inject the heroin under the skin, after which they will get a delayed hit, but at the same time the fix can burn the skin. The dirtier the stuff in the syringe, the more likely it is to burn. And we get some terrible presentations here. Huge soft-tissue infections, big abscesses under the skin affecting arms, forearms, legs . . . eventually they end up with necrotizing fasciitis, which eats away at the skin as you watch.

The other problem with the ward is that all the patients are addicts, otherwise they would not have ended up there, so they have a tendency to abscond. Mostly they will lie in there for a few days, on an antibiotic drip, waiting for the infection to subside slightly, and then as soon as they can, they sneak out of the hospital to score. The prostitutes, of course, end up turning tricks in order to score, so the whole thing can get very seedy indeed. One of the worst things you get asked to do as a junior on that ward is fish out old condoms. The girls often come in and say that the punter had one on but that now she can't find it. In fact it usually transpires, after about twenty minutes of looking, that the punter never had one on at all and had been lying in the first place.

Quite a bit of dealing goes on in the ward too. Mates bring in drugs to sell, and the patients themselves go out to score. Occasionally the situation gets out of control and all the patients get grounded and no one is allowed into or out of the ward. But that only serves to make everyone agitated, and eventually the ward sister relents and then the dealing begins all over again.

Of course, along with all the drug-taking comes the possibility of overdose, and we do occasionally find the odd Hepworth patient dead or in a coma somewhere around the hospital. The favourite places for corpses are the lavatories on the second floor and the stairwell next to the lift. I think we've had about five or six go that way in the last year. One of them was dead at least six hours before anyone noticed her curled up on the stairs.

'What's her name?' asks Ben.

'Nadine,' says the nurse. 'She's mixed race, quite attractive.'

'What, apart from the abscess and the heroin problem,' says Ben.

'You know what I mean,' she says.

'How long ago did you notice her gone?' I ask.

'About fifteen minutes,' she says.

'She could be anywhere by now,' says Ben.

'Actually she hasn't got any shoes on so she can't have gone far,' she replies.

'OK then, you do this floor,' Ben says to the nurse, 'I'll go up, and you can go down,' he adds, looking at me.

'Cheers,' I say, not relishing the idea of looking in the basement.

'Someone's got to check,' he says.

There's something very depressing about wandering around this place in the middle of the night. It's almost as if the hustle and bustle of the hospital prevents you from seeing quite how poorly maintained the actual building is. For all the talk of cleaner hospitals and the desperate desire to combat MRSA, the place is filthy, the toilets are disgusting, and half the building is falling down. The windows are draughty, the roof leaks, and there's mould and damp almost everywhere.

The main problem is that the cleaning staff don't really give a shit. Maybe that's a little strong, but you can understand why they don't feel part of the hospital, or part of our team, because they are not contracted by us. They are contracted out by an agency like Medirest or Sadexo, so I imagine it's hard to feel part of a community where no one speaks to you or even knows your name. The cleaning staff are never invited to any of the parties; no one asks them for a drink in the bar. I imagine they can go through a whole shift, getting paid £6 an hour, without anyone addressing a single word to them.

The problem is that as part of the Private Financial Initiative, where private capital was used to fund public projects such as hospitals, some of the companies that built the new hospitals were given the cleaning contracts as well. The fact that they knew nothing about cleaning hospitals was not an issue; it was a nice little earner to keep them onside. They also, of course, self-regulate. You can always tell when an inspection is coming as the place gets buffed and polished within an inch of its life. Even the swing doors shine.

They are clearly not planning an inspection any time soon, I think as I walk to the stairwell on the ground floor. It smells as if people have been urinating in the corner, which I presume they have.

The same cleaner I saw earlier listening to tunes as he polished the entrance hall floor comes up the stairs towards me. He smells of cigarettes. He looks a little shocked to see someone going down into the basement.

'Excuse me,' I say.

He takes his earphones off.

'Sorry to bother you. I was just wondering if you have seen a woman, a patient, mixed race, come down here?'

He waits for me to finish and doesn't say word.

'A woman? A patient? Down here?'

He clears his throat. He clearly hasn't used his voice for a few hours. 'Je ne comprends rien,' he says, in a thick West African accent. 'I don't understand nothing.' He puts his earphones back on and continues up the stairs.

I walk deeper and deeper into the bowels of the building. It is dark. I can hear the sound of dripping water and the air is cold and damp.

'Hello! Nadine? Are you down here?'

All I hear is my own voice echoing back at me.

Just a few feet away from the stairs there's a pile of broken hospital beds and piles of boxes of what look like IV fluids. They must be out of date otherwise why on earth are they down here?

'Hello!' I shout again.

A scuttling noise comes from the far corner. I'm afraid I don't like the sound very much.

'Nadine?' I try again.

This place is horrible, I think to myself; no one is going to come down here, no matter how desperate they are for a fix. I start to walk up the stairs and for some reason I am spooked slightly and break into a run. I'm quite out of breath by the time I reach the top of the stairs.

Although not as short of breath as the woman panting over her suitcase in the entrance hall.

'My God! You OK?' I ask, running over to her.

She just looks at me. Her face is puce, her cheeks are puffing nineteen to the dozen, her mouth is circular as she inhales and exhales short little breaths. She grabs hold of my hand and gives it a tight squeeze.

'Ahhh!' she says, finally, as she relaxes. 'Jesus! That was a bad one.'

'How far apart are your contractions?'

'Three, four minutes,' she says. 'Not long now.'

'No,' I say, feeling slightly alarmed. 'Anyone else with you?' I look towards the door, expecting a frantic husband to sprint in with more bags, fluffy pillows and a CD player.

'No, just me,' she says, grabbing my hand again, with her left hand. She is wearing a wedding ring. 'I've got two other kids, he's at home with them.'

'Oh. Right.' I pick up her bag for her and put my arm around her very expansive waist. 'Let me get you to Maternity.'

She walks very slowly towards the lift. I look around for a bit more help. Neither of the security guards is anywhere to be seen.

'Are you sure you can do this on your own?'

'I've got my phone,' she huffs. 'I did the last one on my own – oh God!' She turns and grabs my shoulders. 'That huuuuuurts!'

Now I am frightened. I really don't want to deliver this baby in the entrance hall. 'Don't push!' I say.

'I want to!' she yells.

'Well, don't!' I yell right back. 'Let's get you into the lift!'

12–1 a.m.

Fortunately I manage to deposit the labouring Justine at Maternity, but not before she has attempted to squeeze my right hand off, wrench both my shoulders and succeed in peeing on my left shoe. It seemed like we waited an age slumped against the locked door, but fortunately two midwives and a nurse came to my rescue, ushering the lowing Justine to a delivery suite. I did offer to come and hold her hand but she was not keen, and seeing as we had only just met I did not see the point in persisting.

A surprising number of women who have partners deliver babies alone in hospital. Either, like Justine, because they have no one else to look after their children, or their partners can't make it as their labour comes on early and they are at the other end of the country, or things happen too quickly and they arrive only at the last moment. There are of course some women who would rather the father were not there at all. As I stand waiting for the lift with one soggy shoe, I can't help but admire Justine. If that were me in there, I'd want the full drugs menu, as well as gas and air, and a brass band outside trumpeting my marvellousness.

Back down in A&E, Sandra is none too keen on singing my praises. 'Where on earth have you been?' she asks, her steely grey eyes narrowing. We both know she wants to say either 'fuck' or 'hell' in that sentence but is too professional to do so.

I begin with Nadine the prostitute and am about to get on to Justine the mother-to-be when she waves her hand and walks away, like she's dealing with an errant mendacious teenager. I begin to walk after her when I hear a commotion at the doors of A&E.

'Look, I'm dying! I need to see a doctor right now! Do you understand? I am *dying*!'

A man in his early thirties is shouting at the spotty junior on reception, whose name is Kareem – one of our more regular temps. He does eight hours at a time on the front line for about £17,000 a year. Devoid of medical qualifications and only possessing minor secretarial skills, he is responsible for organizing the triage system and therefore the order in which the patients are seen. This, as you can imagine, becomes increasingly difficult and demanding as the night progresses.

Standing next to the screaming man in the suit is a flapping woman in silver high heels and pink silk cocktail dress. 'Jerry, Jerry,' she pleads, 'calm down, you're only making it worse.'

'Worse? How can I be making it worse? I am having a fuck-ing heart attack!' He bends over to the left, clutching his chest.

'I can't breathe! I'm dying! See? Help me!' he begs Kareem.

'OK,' I say, running over to gather Jerry as he collapses on the floor. 'Can you give me a hand?' I ask the girlfriend.

Together we drag Jerry into resus. He is shouting and screaming and grabbing his chest. Ben comes rushing over, as does Stacy. We all get him on to a bed and start taking his clothes off and attaching monitors to him. Jerry's expensive cotton shirt is ripped off him and his leather brogue shoes are chucked on the floor.

'Where does it hurt?'

'What have you been doing tonight, Jerry?'

'Are you allergic to anything?'

'On a scale of one to ten, what is the pain?'

'Jerry?'

'Jerry?'

'Talk to us, Jerry.'

Jerry is getting very pale, his mouth is going blue; he looks from Ben, to me, to Stacy, unable to speak. The heart monitor kicks in. His heart is beating like he's sprinting a bloody marathon. His BP is 160/110. All the alarms are ringing on the machines.

'He's been taking cocaine!' the girl in pink shouts, throwing her hands in the air. 'Two grams, maybe more.'

'Coke?' I say, looking at the heart monitor and Jerry's white face.

Ben riffles through Jerry's suit pocket and pulls out a small white envelope. 'Coke,' he confirms.

'Yes, yes, yes, coke!' repeats the girl, wiping her nose on the back of her hand. 'Is he having a coke stroke?'

'More like a coke-induced heart attack, I'd say,' says Ben, grabbing the ECG machine.

Cocaine accounts for about 25 per cent of all heart attacks in men in their thirties. In some parts of the UK, like ours, as many as one in three strokes or heart attacks in young men is coke-related. And old Jerry here is the perfect example. We need to stabilize his heart, calm him down and stop the irregular beating. The ECG results are not looking good for him, but on the other hand, it's unlikely to be fatal. It's a huge shock to his system but he got here in time and he's young enough to recover. We hope.

'Please don't let him die,' begs the girl. 'Please don't let him die. He's only thirty-three.' She starts to pace the room, rubbing her nose and scratching herself with worry. 'You've got to help him! Hang on in there, Jerry.' It's clear she's been at the coke as well. She sits down and stands up, scratches her arm, scratches the back of her neck, and rubs her nose again and again, while we pump Jerry with more drugs – GTN, morphine – and cover his face with an oxygen mask.

Eventually I shoot Stacy a look to try to get rid of this irritating woman.

'Would you like a cup of tea?' asks Stacy, trying to shift her out of the area.

'Tea?' the girl says, stopping in her tracks. She looks like she is about to retch at the very idea.

'With milk?' adds Stacy.

The girl's shoulders flex involuntarily; she's nearly sick. 'No thanks,' she manages to say as all the saliva drains from her mouth.

Stacy finally extracts her from the room, suggesting that she must have some phone calls to make. She mutters something about Jerry being in capable hands and in the right place, and slowly but surely the girl leaves. The tension automatically dissipates, leaving Ben and me to get on with the job. And by the time Stacy comes back Jerry is breathing a little more normally. The strong drugs are beginning to calm the effects of the cocaine, his arteries are opening, and Jerry's cheeks are pinked up a little.

He opens his eyes and blinks as he takes in the tubes, machines and oxygen mask.

'You'll be OK,' says Stacy, giving his hand a squeeze.

He looks pathetically grateful.

'And your girlfriend is outside calling a few people, including your parents.'

His BP suddenly increases and he breathes heavily into his mask.

Stacy looks at me and then at Jerry. 'Don't worry, there are no visitors allowed in here.'

He looks relieved.

'We'll be sending you up for an angioplasty just as soon as we can track down a consultant.'

'You'll go to the angiography suite for a primary angioplasty,' I explain, 'where they stick a catheter up through the arteries in the groin or wrist and into the heart, to find the blocked artery, and open it up with a stent.'

His eyes widen with terror over the top of his mask. Never before has a man regretted a night out more.

'Don't worry,' I say, slapping the back of his cannulated hand. 'You'll be fine.'

242

I leave Jerry to contemplate minor heart surgery and go and have a piss. I've been desperate to go for a while now and I definitely need a cup of coffee. You tap into your adrenalin when you are dealing with an emergency like Jerry. Your heart beats faster, almost as fast as his, and you concentrate and focus and get through it, riding the wave. It's only when the job's over that you feel a little flat, and now I have to say I feel very tired indeed.

I stand in front of the urinal, trying not to let my head fall forward and hit the wall. I'm wondering if I might slope off for a snooze soon. The next few hours are always the busiest in A&E and then I'm off at three a.m. The end of the graveyard shift. Off back to my flat and a pissed, pissed-off girlfriend. I can't wait.

'You all right?' asks Ben, arriving in the next-door stall. 'That was a bit touch and go.'

'Do you think?' I say, stifling a yawn. 'It was pretty textbook to me. We get quite a few of those in a month. They're normally surrounded by a bit more of an entourage than Timmy.'

'Jerry,' corrects Ben.

'Whatever his name was or is, I am quite tired,' I say, finishing up.

'Well, do you want some of this?' asks Ben, shaking his cock and pulling up his trousers before plucking a white envelope out of his scrubs pocket.

I obviously look a little shocked.

'What?' he says. 'Like he's going to fancy a line in the next twenty-four hours.'

'True,' I say.

'Anyway, it's A&E perks.'

Drugs, like cocaine, heroin and E, are normally confiscated when they come into A&E. Although quite what happens to the drugs when a patient is relieved of their gram, pills or packets is anyone's guess. There's no particular precedent or protocol for patients' drugs; I think everyone just presumes they are destroyed or thrown away, which of course they are. Sometimes. And sometimes they are not. The good stuff gets pocketed and used up elsewhere; the rubbish gets thrown away. The pills tend not to be pinched, because the patients with pills who end up in A&E are, of course, the ones who are having a bad time and who are clearly in possession of some bad gear. The powder is the stuff that goes walkabout. And who can blame us? A cheeky gram here and there. After all, there's nowhere else in the department to put the stuff!

'A small one?' asks Ben, already in the toilet cubicle, chopping one out with his hospital ID card.

I have to admit I am tempted. I am shattered and I could do with a little something to get me through the next couple of hours. But the idea of going back home and having an argument with the drunken Emma when I'm a little wired means I'd lose all the moral high ground. Quite apart from the fact that I have just had to resuscitate someone who's been using this very stuff.

'No thanks,' I say.

'If you're sure,' says Ben, taking a biro out of his top pocket and pulling out the ink tube. He puts the hollow plastic case to his nose and snorts a line of white powder off the loo seat. He gags a tiny bit as the coke hits the back of his nose and throat. 'Urrrh,' he coughs. His eyes water. 'That's good shit.' He looks at me and licks his finger before running it over the top of the loo seat, picking up any residue and rubbing the same finger over his gums. 'Have you ever managed to get your hands on any NHS coke?'

During rhinoplasty, or nose jobs, a substance called Moffat's solution is used, 6 to 10 per cent of which is cocaine, mixed with adrenalin and sodium bicarbonate. It is put up in the nasal lining before the operation to help stem the amount of bleeding. It comes in a pot with two grams' worth of paste in it and any of the solution that is not used is either poured down the sink or thrown in the sharps box. During which time the anaesthetist will announce over and over again, 'I am getting rid of the Moffat's solution, I am not throwing the Moffat's solution in . . .' It's all very worthy and we all have to watch as the potent pick-me-up is thrown away.

'Sadly, no, I haven't.'

'I bet it would blow your head off,' he says, sniffing. 'I had to fill in for someone who was caught pinching drugs when I was training, but he was caught taking diamorphine and diazepam.' He sniffs again as he emerges from the cubicle. 'He was injecting the stuff. It took them over a year to catch him, and when he was finally caught there was no hand-wringing or any of that shit. He was put on four months' leave, he got a rap across the knuckles, and that was that.'

'How did he get caught?'

'It was one of the nurses who finally noticed that Trevor, or whatever his name was, was very keen on the drugs key. They didn't notice when the vials of diamorphine went missing, only that one doc was very helpful when it came to getting supplies for people.'

'I think they are a little tighter here,' I suggest.

'More's the pity,' says Ben. 'I mean, you use the stuff every day, it would be quite nice to have a shot or two. We know how it works, we're hardly going to OD or anything, are we? Just a bit of fun.'

'I can't say I'm too keen on trying that one.'

'Yeah, well, if you hang around here long enough, it's enough to turn anyone to drugs.' He grins. 'Ever thought of chucking it all in and becoming a GP?'

'A GP? My dad's a GP.'

'What? One of those hundred-and-seventy-grand-a-year ones, the ones who "earn more than the Prime Minister"?' he asks, doing the quotation-marks-in-the-air thing.

'Sadly not.'

'I've been looking into it,' announces Ben. 'You know, if the old blow-jobs-for-Botox thing doesn't work out I think I could cope with a life of coughs, colds, chicken pox and the odd bit of housewives' depression. I know it's a fine line between bore-dom and a nice life, but I bet I could tread it.'

'My dad always says that being a GP is ninety-five per cent boredom and five per cent sheer panic.'

'I'd be good at that,' Ben responds. 'I'm a good listener. Did you know that in the US they've worked out that if you let a patient wang on for thirteen minutes they will leave your surgery happy, happy in the knowledge that they have really been listened to. Apparently twelve minutes won't cut it. Only thirteen.'

'Brilliantly we have only five- to ten-minute slots here in the UK. The patient has to be in and out in a maximum of eight minutes for the system to work at its optimum level.'

'That's why everyone always feels so hard done by,' he chuckles. 'But then, all those guys care about is hitting their quality achievement targets and clocking up some "Quality Operation Framework" points, and trousering a nice big fat Billy bonus.'

'I don't think all GPs are that mercenary,' I say.

'Well, they should be,' says Ben. 'It's dog eat dog out there and the government is going to cut through everything like a knife through butter; they're just softening up the public at the moment. They used to want to save all elements of the NHS, but if there's enough briefing against doctors, telling everyone how much we earn all the time, talking about bonuses, then everyone will say "Oh fuck 'em, halve their cash, what do we care?" Mark my words,' he says, tapping the side of his nose. 'Anyway, where do you want to end up?'

'Royal London,' I say. 'Best trauma unit in the country.'

'Yeah,' he nods. 'If you have to get run over, do it just outside the Royal London. If you want to set fire to yourself, do it next to the Northwood, best plastic surgery and burns unit in the country.'

'Give birth?' I ask.

'Oh,' he says, 'that's a hard one. Maybe Tommy's – best view in the country, over the Thames at the Houses of Parliament?'

'Worst place to have an accident?'

'Oh God,' he sniffs. 'So many to choose from. Somewhere shit up north that you've never heard of until they start killing people and then everyone pretends that they're shocked and that they haven't been fiddling their stats for years? God, I remember working in a hospital where we would cancel all operations because we knew someone was coming to inspect the A&E department. We'd stop all operations so that this sod, who must have been in on it too, would say "Isn't it great, there's no waiting for beds, there's no one in the corridors, everything works really well. Here, have some more money and a little performance-related bonus." And then they'd bugger off, we'd start operating again, and there'd be trolleys in the corridors. All sorts of shit.'

'If you don't hit targets, you don't get your money, and if you don't get your money, your hospital withers on the vine – so you have to lie,' I agree.

'Are you sure you don't want a line?' Ben says suddenly. 'I think I fancy another sharpener before going back out there.'

'No, no thanks. But be my guest. I'd better get back out there now, in fact.'

I leave Ben in the toilet to rack up another line and talk to his reflection and go to check on Jerry. Stacy is with him, checking the heart monitor.

'How's the BP?' I ask, checking his chart.

'Down to one twenty over eighty,' she says. 'He seems to be a lot more comfortable.'

'Good. And the girlfriend?'

'She's wearing out a trench, pacing up and down in the waiting room.'

'You should tell her to go. Jerry will be going up soon so she may as well go home.'

'Sure,' she says. 'It's busy out there.'

'It's always busy out there,' I say. 'I suppose I should help Sanjay, Alex and the others out.'

'The two juniors are looking very stressed,' she smiles.

I go over to the computer and pick up another case.

'Mr Richards,' I call. 'Mr Richards?'

Two men, one middle-aged and the other quite elderly, come towards me. The older man, wearing split working-men's boots and an overcoat tied with string, looks a little disoriented. It looks like he's been sleeping rough. The younger man is much better dressed. I sit them both down together in a cubicle and start to take notes. It transpires that the older man is the younger man's father and has been missing for two years. The father has a history of mental health problems and has just turned up out of the blue at his son's house. I nod and listen to the story. I ask the old boy all the requisite questions to see if he is on the ball. What day is it today? The date? His name? The name of the Prime Minister? He gets them all correct except the name of the Prime Minister, but I have to say that flummoxes quite a few people these days. He doesn't appear to be suicidal. I check him over briefly, and he's not ill either. So I share the good news with the son that his father is fine and can go home.

The son starts to get cross. He wants me to admit his father.

'I'm afraid I can't,' I say. 'I have no grounds to admit him. He is well.'

'But he has mental health problems,' says the son, beginning to raise his voice.

'Not at the moment.'

'He's had them before.'

'Not now he hasn't.'

'But he's crazy!'

'Not now he isn't,' I insist.

'OK, well, we don't want him at home with us!' he shouts. 'The man's got nits. I don't want him to give them to my kids.'

'I'm sorry, sir, but this is not a drop-in centre for the elderly, nor is it a place for you to dump members of your family because it is inconvenient for you to look after them. If you want to dump your father, then I'm afraid you need to take him to Social Services in the morning and perhaps they can arrange for him to be housed elsewhere. We can't look after him here. This is a place for accidents and emergencies, and your father is neither.'

Perhaps I should have been a little more tactful, but I found his callousness in front of his own father rather shocking.

'You fucking racist!' he shouts at me. 'Just because I'm black.'

'It has got nothing to do with the fact that you are black, Mr Richards. Black or white, I am not admitting somebody into hospital unless they are ill.'

'YOU! ARE! A FUCKING RACIST!' He is really shouting now, jabbing his finger at me, and I can feel my heart pounding. It is not a pleasant experience. 'I want your name! Give me your name! Give me your name! I am going to report you!'

I am not obliged to give him my name, and the last thing I want is him coming after me. So I refuse. This, of course, pisses him off even more.

Finally, Sandra arrives to try to defuse the situation. Mr

Richards Jr fills her in on my supposed racism and the fact that I refused to give my name.

'I'm sorry, sir, but you need to calm down,' Sandra says. 'Or I will have to call security.'

Unlike some hospitals, where emergency staff wear ripcord alarms around their waists that they can pull in the event of their being threatened, we have nothing here. And even when security does arrive they can't do anything; they can't touch a member of the public unless that person has actually been physically abusive towards us. Punters can stand there and verbally abuse you for fifteen, twenty, thirty minutes at a time, indeed as long as they like, and no one can do anything about it.

Mr Richards does not calm down, and it takes about five minutes for the two sleepy security officers to arrive. They are about as effective as a fart in a wind tunnel. Mr Richards carries on shouting at me for the next quarter of an hour while a concerned crowd gathers. Some try to reason with him, others just keep telling him to calm down, but he is not listening. He keeps on shouting and I just stand there and take it. Eventually, when I realize that he is not going to stop and the security guards are not going to do anything for fear of being sued, I give up.

'Here,' I say, 'here's my name.' I write it down on a piece of paper. 'And now, can you please leave me alone!'

251

1–2 a.m.

I have to say, now is about the time I wish I had a hip flask in the changing room. After being on the end of an aggressive finger-jabbing tirade like that, you kind of want a few minutes on your own and a shot or two to calm your nerves. Not that Mr Richards is the worst I've ever had. I have been hit with a clipboard, punched in the back, and kicked in the stomach as I tried to restrain a drug addict who was chucking stuff around and threatening members of staff.

Despite all the last government initiatives and clampdowns and £1,000 fines, the level of violence inflicted on us is increasing. One in ten NHS workers has been physically abused on the job; nearly one in five of us has been verbally harassed or bullied. Nurses and doctors have had knives pulled on them; they've been punched in the face, seriously beaten up, even sexually assaulted. And no amount of training, or courses, or talks can prepare you for someone who is suddenly going to lash out or get violent. Ambulance crew and staff working with mental health patients or those with severe learning disabilities are obviously more at risk, but a drunk schoolteacher is just as likely to hit you in the face as a crackhead who's been picked up off the street. There are no standards any more. I have to say it's one of the most unpleasant aspects of the job. If anything is going to make me pack it all in and open a beach bar in Thailand, or indeed go into the private sector, it's that.

Without a shot of vodka to calm my slightly jangled system, I decide to go outside and have a cigarette. As I walk out of the department, Sandra catches my eye. I half expect her to call me back, but she doesn't. I suspect she would like to come along too, if only she smoked. It was quite intense in that cubicle, and it was actually thanks to her that Mr Richards finally left, taking his poor, confused, tired old dad with him. What sort of welcome home is that, I wonder as I walk down the stairs to the car park. Poor bloke. He's been two years on the streets and has finally found his way home, only for his son to try to dump him on us.

We do get quite a bit of Granny Dumping, as it is called in A&E, but more usually towards Christmas. Carers who have had enough and want to go out on the razzle turn up with an old girl, explain that she's had a fall, or a turn, or a tumble, and we are obliged to take her in for the night for observation. Even if the old person denies what has happened, the carer will argue that they are suffering some sort of dementia and the old person can't remember what has happened to them in the last three minutes let alone in the last three hours. The carer then runs for the hills or the nearest bar, only to come back the next day to collect the elderly person, nursing a rather rough hangover. And those are the nice ones. We get some who dump and run. They take their poor unsuspecting parent by the hand, lead them into A&E and walk straight out. These are the really bad cases, where the old person does actually have dementia and doesn't even know their own name, their address or the phone number of their nearest but perhaps not so dearest. We usually manage to trace these people through some route or another, but it's depressing and it's hard work. There is something deeply callous about dumping someone so old and frail and vulnerable. What these people don't seem to realize is that they will be the same one day. Let's hope their own children will be a little more forgiving.

Standing outside smoking my cigarette, I suddenly shiver with cold, like someone has walked over my grave. I must be tired. It's all these morbid thoughts I'm having. It's enough to make anyone miserable.

I can hear the click-clack of heels coming towards me out of the darkness. I watch as an attractive thirtysomething woman comes towards me. She's not walking in a particularly straight line; she is certainly out of it. She pauses in the car park and looks around. Although I am quite close by, she doesn't appear to see me. She stops between two cars and starts to take her clothes off. She whips off her top and short skirt and then rummages around in an orange Sainsbury's bag. As she takes her bra off and puts on a patient's gown that she pulls out of the bag, it suddenly dawns on me who she is.

'Nadine?' I shout.

She turns around, looking confused, unsure of where the sound came from.

'Nadine?'

She squints over at me. 'Who wants to know?'

'Are you Nadine? From Hepworth Ward?'

'I might be,' she says.

'Well, they're looking for you.'

'They are?' She sounds slightly alarmed. 'Who is?'

'One of the nurses.'

'Oh,' she replies, looking completely nonplussed. 'Well, I'm here now, aren't I?'

She walks towards me in her high heels and patient's gown. It's a rather incongruous combination to say the least. 'Have you got a fag?' she asks, looking at me intently. Her pupils are like tiny pinpricks. She's high as a kite.

I pull a Silk Cut out of my packet and give to her.

'Got anything stronger than that?' she asks.

'No.'

'Oh.'

She takes the cigarette. Her arms are covered in bandages and strapping. I half expect her to lean in for a light. But she doesn't. She takes the fag and pops it behind her ear.

'See you later,' she smiles, and heads for the side door.

It's locked. You need a swipe key to get in.

'Can you open this?' she says.

I go over to let her in. She smiles again, and in the light of the stairwell I can tell that she was once a very pretty girl. But now her skin is dull, her eyes have no focus and some of her teeth are black.

She turns and walks slowly up the stairs.

I finish my cigarette and throw the butt into the car park, to join my ever-growing pile. What I wouldn't give for a few Treat and Street, or a quick turnaround of patients, now just to keep me occupied before I clock off at three a.m.

Back in A&E I bump into Ben, who is just coming out of a cubicle.

'You OK?' he asks.

'Not too bad. You?'

'Fucking hell, you should see the beast I've got in there. Tooth to tattoo ratio is not good.' He shakes his head.

I smile. I haven't heard that phrase in a while. A positive ratio of more teeth than tattoos is shorthand for ascertaining the IQ of the patient. More tats than teeth and you are fucked.

'What's he done?'

'Brained himself in a fight, obviously,' he says. 'It's a simple stitch-up, that's all.'

Beyond Ben, the place is heaving. Sanjay is flapping out an X-ray, Alex has a load of bloods in his fist, Stacy is walking an old bloke to a cubicle, there are a couple of juniors in other cubicles coping with some drunks, and Ian is still here.

'No home to go to?' I say.

'Nor do you,' he replies.

'But I'll be paid extra.'

'And I have nothing better to do,' he smiles. I must look like I believe him, so he laughs. 'No, I'm waiting for Mr Armstrong to finish up.'

'Is he still here as well?'

'He's just doing some final checks on Mr Hughes, checking

his bowels have not been perforated by the vibrator, and then I think he and I are going off for a nightcap somewhere.'

'What, alcohol?' Weirdly, my mouth starts to salivate, it sounds so tempting.

'I know plenty of places where you can get a few brandies at two a.m.,' he says, tapping the side of his nose. 'You can join us if you'd like.'

'I'd love to, but I've got a drunk girlfriend waiting for me at home.'

'Oh God.' His nose crinkles in disgust. I'm not sure if it's the word 'drunk' or 'girlfriend' that's putting him off so much. 'If I were you I'd sleep here. Let her sober up and deal with her in the morning.'

'Here?'

'There are plenty of beds,' he shrugs.

I amble over to the computer, thinking about Ian's suggestion. It's not a bad idea. It could possibly be a good solution to a tricky problem. Let her sleep it off and go back home when she's gone to work. That way we'd avoid any confrontation, and quite frankly I don't have the energy for an argument.

I walk out into the waiting room. It now smells properly of alcohol and old sweat. I call out the next name on the list and a Mr Lundy gets off his chair and starts to shuffle towards me. In his sixties, dressed in a macintosh, with thick glasses, he appears neither drunk nor like he is having a heart attack. I am slightly wondering why he is here. I sit him down in a cubicle and take his details.

'Now, how can I help you?' I ask.

'It's my head,' he starts. 'It's hurting.'

My heart sinks. There is nothing worse than a headache in the middle of the bloody night. Of all the presentations to wish for, this is one of the worst. It sounds so simple but it's a bloody nightmare. A stomach ache is fine. So much more bog standard. You have a feel around, there are certain things you can rule in or out, you can do a quick ultrasound if you are worried. But with a head, there are so many things it could be, from a full-blown brain tumour to just a touch of dehydration. What you really want to do is kick awake the radiology consultant and get your patient a CT scan, but they will only do that in an emergency and more often than not your patient does not fit the criteria. You need a blown pupil or blood coming out of the nose or eyes before anyone will so much as answer the phone.

The more I listen to Mr Lundy, the more alarm bells start to ring. He tells me his wife has terminal lung cancer and he's been looking after her for the past eleven months. She hasn't got long left. She's asleep at the moment, which is why he's come in the middle of the night; he doesn't have time in the day. His headaches have been bothering him for a few months now; he gets double vision and excruciating pain. He's been stealing a few of his wife's painkillers, but the pain is now becoming unbearable.

'So, on a scale of one to ten, with ten being the most painful, how bad is your headache now?'

'Um, eight?' he says, moving his head gingerly, his left eye flickering with pain.

We both know he means ten, but I jot down his rating anyway.

I have seen this happen quite often in elderly patients, where one is ill and the other is caring for them. The carer starts to feel unwell but does nothing about it because they don't have time, and then when they finally get round to it they don't present until it is far too late.

'Well, I'll tell you what we'll do,' I say, with a smile, 'we'll give you something for the pain and I'll have a word and see if we can have a look inside that head of yours.' I write 'Vit M' down on his file – Vitamin M, or morphine – and go to find Ian to try and work out my chances of getting Mr Lundy scanned here and now.

Ian is sympathetic enough for a bloke who's worked a twelve-hour shift and is desperate for a drink at half one in the morning, but he tells me what I already know: Mr Lundy needs to go home, make an appointment with his GP and get himself referred in the hope that there is an appointment available for him within the next five or six weeks. And he also needs to hope that whatever it is that's going on inside his head does not get any bigger or badder between now and then.

By the time I'm back with Mr Lundy, Stacy's administered the shot of morphine and he seems to look a little less agonized. I think the fact that I haven't taken one look at him and immediately wanted to cut his head open has cheered him up a little – that and, perhaps, the fact that someone else is looking after him for a change.

'I will be all right, though, won't I, doctor?' he asks. 'Because my wife needs me.'

I have no idea if he'll be fine or not, but the symptoms aren't stacking in his favour. He is the wrong side of fifty, and he's got a stinking headache that he says he's had for a while, and that makes me think he's probably had it for at least six months. But instead of saying what I really think, I decide to lie.

I hate doing it. I remember a few months back being with a woman who had pancreatitis and had just had a pancreatico-duodenectomy, and all she kept on asking me was when she could go home, and all I could think was 'I know you're not leaving this place, unless you go out feet first.' But you can't say that. You can't tell someone who still has a bit of hope in their eyes that they are going to die. It's cruel. Equally, it's not so brilliant to lie. So you say things like 'Well, you still need our help a bit.' Or 'Maybe just a couple more weeks.' Or 'You're doing very well, let's see what happens in the next couple of days.' Then they start to deteriorate, and then they stop asking when they are leaving and start concentrating on the battle at hand.

And it is a battle. Sometimes you can almost see and hear death approaching. You can certainly smell it. There is a sweet odour of putrefaction that suddenly sets in. Like the person has turned, and you know it won't be long. The air around them becomes heavy, and, oddly, the human survival instinct means that you don't want to stay with them long. I'm sure that stems back to the time when to stay with the sick and dying meant you too might end up sick and dying. It's certainly true that when patients are close to death you want to be with them less. It's an urge that as a doctor you learn to fight. They also seem to turn away from the light. They engage less, they refuse visitors who are not completely necessary; needy friends are often turned away.

And of course we help them on their way. To say that we don't assist patients who are dying to go more comfortably or quickly would be a lie. We do. And often. The old Brompton Cocktail is still in existence – a fatal mixture of cocaine, morphine and, in the old days, gin. The Brompton Cocktail was originally used in the 1920s to allow terminally ill patients to have a less painful death. Pioneered at the Royal Brompton for patients with tuberculosis, hence the name, it was originally the idea of Dr Herbert Snow, who had first thought of helping the terminally ill on their way in the late 1890s. These days we just up the morphine in their drip. It's one of those great unsaids within the hospital system. There's never much chat about what's going on. You instruct the nurse to up the morphine, which causes respiratory arrest; she tells you that the respiratory rate is falling, you nod; she says that the rate is now down to less than twelve and that you should do something to reverse the effects, and you nod again and walk on by. With any luck it's over quickly. The patient doesn't fight too long and hard and they are at peace. At last.

'I hope you feel a little better,' I say to Mr Lundy. 'And make sure you make an appointment with your GP first thing tomorrow morning.'

'I will be OK, though, won't I?' he asks again.

'Just make the appointment,' I say, leaving the room. 'I shall leave you in Stacy's capable hands.'

I'm feeling very jaded. I suppose it's because I was thinking about a nice Treat and Street case; I was just after something a little less emotional. Some stitches maybe. Or a drunk. As I reach the computer I look across and see Alex walking another weaving, listing pisshead towards a cubicle. Oh God, I think, rubbing my eyes and rolling my stiff shoulders, only another hour to go.

'Jason Grove?' I shout into a waiting room full of increasingly bizarre-looking people. Underneath the cold strip lights, their evening outfits, the cropped tops, the heels and the smudged make-up look bright and lurid. Another collection of drinking injuries.

I look across at Jason Grove, who is walking towards me like some paranoid, twitching freak. He is white-faced, hollow-cheeked, and his eyes are red-rimmed. The man is clearly in need of cocoa and a good night's sleep.

'Oh thank God, finally,' says a rather plump young woman who is accompanying him. 'We've been waiting ages.'

'Sorry,' I lie. I am beyond caring. 'Follow me.'

Jason is behaving like some cowering idiot. The door is scary. The nurses are scary. The cubicle is clearly an awful place.

'Don't tell me – LSD?' I suggest, double-clicking my pen and rolling my eyes slightly.

'Meow meow,' says Jason, his eyes narrowing, scratching his sandy-blond stubbled chin. 'Meow meow,' he repeats manically. 'Meow meow.'

I'm afraid I am slightly at a loss as to what to do. I look across at the plump girlfriend for some sort of enlightenment.

'He's been up for three days,' she offers.

'Three?'

'Yup,' she nods, despairingly. 'He works in a bank.'

'What, as a trader?'

'No, a cashier,' she says, looking at me like I'm a dick.

'How much has he done?'

'Six,' she says.

'Lines?'

'Grams,' she corrects.

That sounds a lot. But I'm not sure. I have heard of meow meow but I haven't come across it before. It's clearly a stimulant, otherwise Jason wouldn't still be awake. The delusions and paranoid outlook may well be the result of both his lack of sleep and the drug, or just the lack of sleep. Six grams sounds like quite a lot though. Six grams of coke is certainly a lot. Meow meow must be similar.

'Right, back in a tick,' I say. I need to find Ben, or Ian, or someone who knows about this shit.

Thankfully, I bump straight into Ben.

'Meow meow?' I ask.

'What?' he asks keenly. He's looking a little bit wired himself.

'Meow meow?' I ask again.

'What, the drug so good they named it twice?'

'It is what?'

'Fuck knows,' he replies. 'It's a plant fertilizer, mephedrone – a bloke's got standards!' He smiles. 'I did hear the other day that some teenager ripped his own bollocks off after eighteen hours on the stuff.'

'That's not what I call a good night out.'

'I agree,' he laughs.

'Benzo?' I venture.

'Benzo,' he agrees.

Stacy is with Jason when I get back. It seems he's managed to rip a whole load of paper off the giant paper roll we use to cover each trolley, and thrown some equipment around. He's also now convinced that he's covered in centipedes, and he has a nosebleed. It has exploded down the front of his T-shirt, but he can't sit still enough to stem the flow of blood because he keeps tearing at his own creeping crawling flesh with his fingernails.

'Hurry up!' the girlfriend shrieks at me. 'You've got to do something!'

2–3 a.m.

A great big dose of the sedative, hypnotic, anticonvulsant and muscle relaxant benzodiazepine does the trick and Jason finally gives up on scratching at the imaginary bugs crawling all over him and goes to sleep. He is taken upstairs for observation in case of seizures, more nosebleeds, or indeed scratching himself stupid.

As he disappears off towards the lift with his fat-thighed girlfriend in tow, I see Mr Lundy disappearing off into the night to continue looking after his extremely sick wife. I can't help thinking, as I watch him shuffle away, that we've got this system wrong. A fuckwit can stay up for three days, willingly shoving plant fertilizer or whatever up his nose, and expect us to gather him up with open arms when he can no longer deal with the consequences of it all. But an old boy who has been nursing his wife for nearly a year comes for our help and gets shunted off with an appointment card and the possibility of a six-week wait for a CT scan he needs but which I can't order up because he doesn't meet the criteria. The sad thing is, both he and I know there is possibly something rather large and malignant inside his skull and there is probably very little we can do about it.

Sanjay walks past me with a large IV bag full of luminous green liquid. 'Have you seen the drop-in centre we're running?' he asks, indicating the other side of the room where three men are lined up in a row, each with a bag of Pabrinex hanging next to them.

'Bloody hell.'

'I know,' nods Sanjay. 'And there's another one about to join them. It's drunk night tonight. The tramps must be having a party.'

It's an odd sight, three of them sitting in a row, attached to their vitamin B drips, chatting away – in so much as full-blown fall-down-drunk alcoholics can chat. Most alcoholics are vitamin B deficient, which leads to Wernicke's encephalopathy, or wet brain, a condition that results in short-term memory loss. This is often left untreated, and recent reports suggest that alcohol-related memory loss could account for between 10 and 24 per cent of dementia cases. So it's hard to begrudge them their treatment, but at the same time you can't help thinking that perhaps there are better ways of dealing with the nation's pissheads than patching them up and moving them on. Although I suppose there's only so much we can do with the number of people we have working here and the money available.

'RTA on its way,' announces Sandra, looking at me.

'I'm ready.' I smile at her, attempting to thaw the icicles in her heart. 'Drunk driver?'

'I presume,' she agrees.

A few minutes later the doors slam open and two green paramedics come running in, pushing a trolley at high speed. Alex rushes over to join me. We both lean over the gurney expecting to see a mutilated, mashed, bloodied face. Or at least a smashed-open chest, where the steering wheel has gone through, plus a couple of mutilated limbs and some random intestines. Instead, there's a rather attractive twentysomething female wearing an oxygen mask and a neck brace, giggling her head off.

'Her name's Vicky,' says the lanky member of the ambulance crew. 'She's twenty-three and rolled her Clio off the road.'

At which the girl shrieks with laughter. We all look at her.

'She's been like this since we picked her up,' shrugs lanky bloke.

'Shock?' I suggest.

'Or a nutter,' he whispers in my ear.

'Yes,' I nod. 'Or indeed one of those.'

'OK then, Vicky,' says Alex, 'does it hurt anywhere? Can you feel and move all your limbs?'

Vicky carries on laughing.

'Well, she's certainly consistent, I'll give her that,' I say. 'On four. One, two, three, four!'

Alex, Stacy and I lift Vicky off the stretcher and on to the bed. This only serves to delight her even more.

'She seems fine to me,' says Stacy.

'If somewhat hysterical,' I say.

267

'We're going to have to check her over,' says Alex, taking a small torch out of his pocket to check her pupils. 'She is effectively non-responsive.'

'The full trauma handshake?' I say, so-called because almost every RTA gets a finger up the arse when they come into A&E. It's standard procedure, to see if the spinal cord is intact. You put a finger up their backside, ask them to clench their buttocks, and if they can then all systems are go.

'Don't worry, I'll do that,' says Alex, pulling rank.

'Fine by me,' I say. I can't think of anything worse.

Sandra cuts off Vicky's trousers and we roll her over. She is now laughing uncontrollably. I'm beginning to think it's a mixture of shock and embarrassment that has set her off. Alex slaps me on the leg and gestures for me to look at Vicky's rather nice backside. She's wearing a G-string with the words 'Kiss My Arse' written across the top. Alex winks and grins before snapping on his rubber gloves.

'Now I'm sorry, Vicky, but we have to do this, just to check that you haven't really hurt yourself. As part of a bones and joints check we need to do the spinal column, and that means a rectal exam. So I will put my finger up your backside and then I want you to clench – OK?'

Vicky squeals with laughter and nods her head.

'OK then, Vicky, here we go.'

Alex's hand moves up between Vicky's legs and between her buttocks. She suddenly falls silent.

'And clench!' orders Alex. 'Clench, Vicky!'

'I'm sorry,' says Vicky rather quietly, turning around to look at Alex, 'but I think you've got the wrong hole.'

'Sorry! Oh my God, have I? I can only apologize!'

I have never seen a man move his hand more quickly or his face blush so profoundly in my life. Alex withdraws from the cubicle at speed, muttering under his breath, 'I think you'd better finish up here.'

It turns out that Vicky is completely fine. She managed to roll her car three times and write it off, but because she was only going at about 7 mph and due to the large amount of Baileys in her system, she came to no harm. Her Clio was a write-off, but she is completely fine. Alex, on the other hand, is so mortified that he has to take himself off for a few minutes in order to calm himself down.

'I can't believe I just did that,' he says, pacing up and down in the corridor outside.

'It's an easy mistake to make,' says Ben, joining us.

'Well, not really,' says Alex. 'One hole is fairly distinct from the other.'

'She didn't seem to mind,' I add, trying to be helpful.

'She probably enjoyed it!' encourages Ben. 'I remember when I was very junior a consultant asked me to do a pelvic on a rather large Afro-Caribbean lady. She was there, legs akimbo, and the consultant kept on saying to me, "Can you feel the uterus? Can you feel the cervix?" And after about five minutes of sweating and prodding and poking, the woman pops her head up off the bed and shouts, "Boy! You carry on like that and you are going to ring my bell!"'

'That was quite clearly the end of your obs and gynae career,' I laugh.

'I made a large lady very happy!' he laughs.

'Well, I suppose it's only marginally worse than the rectal I did the other day,' says Alex. 'This old biddy had a swollen abdomen and I had to pop the finger in. I rolled her over, and as it went in she said, "Oh, Gerald! Is that you?"'

'Jesus Christ!' laughs Ben.

'I had to apologize and say sorry, I wasn't Gerald,' says Alex. 'And all I could think of was "Gerald, you dirty bugger!"'

'Quite literally,' I add.

'Exactly!' he agrees, and then yawns loudly. 'I think I need a cup of coffee. I am actually asleep on my feet.'

'I've done that before,' says Ben.

'What?' I ask.

'Fallen asleep on my feet. You can actually do it. You've just got to get the balance right.' He starts to demonstrate. 'You have this hunch when you get your centre of gravity and you don't need anything to support you and you stand and sleep. And you can make it look like you are looking at the op. I used to do it when I was training, helping someone operate, or sitting down doing surgery in the middle of the night. It just means you are a little slow to hand things over to them. They just ask you twice.'

Watching Ben laugh at his own joke, throwing his nose back to reveal a small lump of coke still lodged in his right nostril, I am struck by how much this profession has changed over the past few years. Ben is old-school. He is bright and charming and funny and quite likely to help himself to the contents of the pharmacy. And he is also a good doctor. But the system doesn't like people like him so much any more. They like the dull wads who put in the time and clock off when they're supposed to.

They don't think laterally, they have never worked out how to sleep standing up, and I think, bizarrely, our profession will suffer as a result. Maybe it's because I'm tired and beginning to get a little emotional at the thought of leaving this place, but I think the system needs a few Bens around to make it take risks and come up with interesting solutions to everyday problems. Otherwise things will just remain static.

'A young woman, pelvic bleeding?' says Sandra, poking her long thin nose through the double doors.

Alex looks at me, and I look at Ben.

'OK then,' I say, 'I'll do it.'

A few minutes later I find myself in a cubicle with Shannon, a pair of rubber gloves and her two mates. We have been trained to be especially sensitive when it comes to young women and pelvic examinations. Normally these are done with a female nurse present to try to minimize any stress and embarrassment, and they are also instructed to talk to the woman afterwards about any fears they have about what the doctor has said. These three, however, are treating the whole thing like some sort of cocktail party.

'All right then, doc?' says one of the friends, who introduces herself as Debbie.

'I'm fine, thanks,' I say, before trying to talk Shannon through the procedure.

'Yeah, yeah, yeah,' she replies, before getting on the bed and pulling up her skirt.

'Steady on there, Shan,' laughs her other mate, who tells me while chomping away on her chewing gum that her name is Grace.

I'm not sure if it's nerves or bravado or both, but these girls are acting strangely. Their friend appears to be having a miscarriage and none of them seems to be taking it at all seriously. I ask the girls to leave the room before I examine their friend but they all insist, including Shannon, on staying. This is the first time I have done a pelvic with an audience, expect when I was a student of course, when the poor patient had to put up with a couple of amateurs rooting around her ovaries in the name of education.

'Ouch,' says Grace, helpfully, as I start.

'Cheers,' giggles Shannon. 'There's no need to look right up my fanny, Grace!'

'Oh my God!' adds Debbie, covering her mouth with her hands. 'He's right up there!'

'Shut it, you two,' smirks Shannon. 'I'm concentrating!'

Thankfully, it doesn't take me long to be able to confirm what I think we all knew, that Shannon is having a miscarriage.

'Yeah, thanks, doc,' she nods from the bed. 'I thought as much.' She appears neither upset nor bothered. She's young, nineteen years old, maybe she's relieved.

'The worst of it appears to be over,' I continue, scanning her young face for any kind of reaction.

Her hair is scraped back tightly off her pale freckled forehead. She has about fifteen studs in her right ear, decreasing in size as they ascend the lobe, like a lesson in perspective. She has long square-tipped fingernails which are painted different colours and covered in tiny diamond studs. I can't help but think if she took as much care over herself as she does her nails, she might not be in this position.

'Telling me!' she laughs with her mates. 'It's been killing me all afternoon.'

'I said you should of come in earlier!' chomps Grace, wagging another bejewelled fingernail. 'I told her she should of,' she says to me.

'Yes, you should have,' I say. 'If only to make sure everything was OK. Did you know how many weeks pregnant you were?'

She looks at me like I've asked her to split the atom. 'Seven? Eight? Nine? Ten?'

'Eleven? Twelve? Thirteen?' laughs Debbie.

'When was the date of your last period?' I ask.

'How should I know!'

'Well, you'd probably know better than me,' I say, beginning to get a little irritated. If she didn't care what was happening to her, why should I?

'Eight, nine weeks ago, I think. Do you know when your last period was, Debs?'

'Me?' says Debs. 'No idea! How about you, Grace?'

'Now!' she laughs. She throws her head back so hard she nearly chokes on her gum.

'Anyway, as I said, I think the worst is over so I think it's probably best if you take yourself back home, then come back to Outpatients in the morning just to make sure everything's OK,' I continue, ignoring their laughter.

'Hey, doc,' says Grace. 'You on Facebook?'

'Sorry?'

'Are you though? On Facebook?'

'Yeah, are you, doc?' asks Shannon, sitting up and pulling her skirt back down.

'Um, yes, I am, but—' I'm not sure I should have said that.

'Wicked!' says Shannon, getting off the bed. 'We'll look you up.'

'Um, well, that's probably not a good idea—'

'Why not?' asks Grace, picking her handbag up off the floor.

'Yeah, chill out, doc,' adds Debbie. 'It might never happen.'

'That your name?' asks Grace, checking the ID card that's clipped to the top of my scrubs trousers. She's a little sharper than the shouting Mr Richards, I'll give her that.

'Um, yes.'

'Excellent,' she says.

'Thanks, doc,' says Shannon, pulling her pants up and then slapping me on the back.

'Do you want anything for the pain?' I ask, as she appears to be on the point of walking straight out of the door.

'No thanks,' she says. 'I've got Solpadeine at home.'

'If you're sure.'

'Cheers,' she says, and she and her mates move straight off down the corridor.

I stand and watch and listen to them giggle their way to the double doors. I don't know whether to be shocked or depressed. I can't help wondering what has happened to those girls for them to be laughing and chatting as their friend is having a miscarriage. Maybe I'm just sentimental, or overtired, and maybe their reaction is more healthy. Nature is a wasteful creature. As many as one in seven pregnancies ends in early miscarriage; maybe we should take these things a little more in our stride. She obviously didn't want the child. And why should she? She's a nineteen-year-old girl with her whole life

ahead of her. But some emotion, some regret, some acknowledgement of what was happening would have actually made it
a little easier for me.

I let the irony of that thought linger in my head.

Suddenly the swing doors slam open and three paramedics
come sprinting towards me. Their faces are determined, their
expressions are grim, and they really are moving very fast.

'Male, twentysomething years old!' he yells at me. 'Machete
attack!'

Who the fuck attacks someone with a machete?

Bang! The doors slam again. Another trolley comes careering towards me with another three paramedics looking equally
focused.

'Male, twentysomething years old!' they yell at me.
'Machete attack!'

The whole department drops what they are doing; soon
there's a sea of nurses, doctors, drips and machines being
pulled and pushed everywhere. The first bloke is squealing and
weeping and shrieking. His body has been sliced all over the
place; there is blood and open flesh everywhere. It's like something out of a hideous slasher movie. The second bloke on the
stretcher is making a sort of low moaning noise; his arms have
been sliced, particularly across the front of his forearms where
he's had his hands up trying to protect his face. They have both
been subjected to one of the most horrific attacks I have ever
seen.

Ben and Alex take the screamer. They tube him and secure
his airways, then line up all the machines and shift him across.
As they move him he lets out a piercing wail that sends shivers

down my spine. Sanjay and I have the other bloke. We tube him and secure his airways too, then Sanjay says, 'On the count of three we move him. One, two, three!' We all lift him up off the stretcher and roll him as quickly and as neatly as we can on to the bed. Stacy rushes around attaching him to all the monitors and I yell out an order for O neg.

'Stop!' shouts Sanjay, his arm raised in the air.

We stop in our tracks, and he points back across to the stretcher. There, in the middle of the stretcher, where the young man's head had been, is his brain. A whole brain. We all stare. Sanjay rolls the dead man over. The whole of the back of his skull has been sliced off. I look at the cavity, then I look at the brain, and then I'm afraid I throw up all over my shoes.

3–4 a.m.

We are all so shocked that none of us speaks for several minutes. I stand there rooted to the spot, my arms hanging by my side, warm vomit seeping slowly into my shoes. Sanjay just scratches his head. No one calls the death. All Stacy can do is stare at the brain, her whole body shaking in disbelief. Even the other well-seasoned members of the team are knocked off their stride. Ben mumbles some profanity, and Alex drops his scissors.

I'm not usually this squeamish. It takes a lot to make me sick, and I have seen a whole human brain many times before – I've even dissected one. So it's not the brain itself that set me off. I think it was the speed of it all. The idea that we had a living breathing man with us one second, then a second later we're left with a corpse and a brain sitting on a stretcher. It's like someone took the batteries out. Flipped the switch. One moment he was moaning, the next he was dead.

'Um, time of death,' says Sanjay, eventually, 'three zero three a.m. OK, let's get him out of here. Amazing,' he adds, turning to have another look at the back of the skull like the true and proper scientist he is. 'I have never seen a skull sliced off like that. Have you?'

'Only in a film,' I reply, slightly less keen on closer inspection.

'It must have been a hell of a blow,' he adds, tracing the line of the skull with his fingertip. 'I know how hard it is to crack open a skull, I've stood in on brain surgery.'

Four policemen arrive in A&E. It's like some police merry-go-round here today. No sooner have SO19 gone upstairs with their gangland shooters than they are replaced by another load of coppers clogging up the doorways, asking questions.

According to the police, these two sliced and diced bodies are the results of a group of Lithuanians having an argument. One of them got a machete and started to attack the other two, before leaving them for dead. The one who is still alive apparently got on his hands and knees and dragged himself along the pavement to the local pub, where he managed to wake the landlord and raise the alarm. He tried very hard to save his friend.

'Poor sod,' said one of the coppers, taking a look at the dead young man on the bed next to us. 'So, how did he die? Loss of blood?'

'No, his brain fell out of the back of his head,' says Sanjay, pointing to the brain still sitting on the stretcher.

The policeman looks across, just to make sure that Sanjay is joking. As soon as he clocks the brain sitting there, still warm and pink, he passes out. His legs fold under him and he hits the floor with an almighty thump, taking a tray of instruments with him.

'I thought they were trained for this sort of thing,' says Sanjay, leaping forward to help the man.

'No one is trained for that,' I say.

'I suppose so,' says Sanjay, feeling the policeman's pulse. 'Did he hit his head? Did you hit your head?' he repeats as the policeman starts to come round.

The policeman mumbles something in reply.

'Put your head between your legs and breathe slowly.' Sanjay looks up at Sandra, who is standing there wondering why her department has been reduced to this chaos. 'Sister, could you make this man some sweet tea?'

'Leave him to me,' she says, bending over and putting a slim arm around the policeman's shoulders. 'Get up, in your own time,' she says. 'And come this way.'

I have to admit that a cup of sweet tea is exactly what I need. I should really be going home. It's the end of the graveyard shift and I am entitled to bugger off. But my shoes are covered in vomit and I am feeling quite out of sorts. Also, the drunken Emma is not exactly a siren beckoning me on to the rocks. I squelch my way into the common room and flick the kettle on.

'Ooh, you read my mind,' says an anaesthetist called Sally as she breezes into the room rubbing her hands. 'I have just been at the best operation,' she says as she bustles around looking for milk in the fridge.

I don't know her that well but I've always found her efficient short hair and tight, pleased smile more than a little annoying.

'It was the smoothest wake-up I have ever done. Literally the man just woke up and opened his eyes. No coughing, or spluttering, or teeth chattering. Nothing. It was a perfect ten out of ten, even though I say it myself.'

'Good,' I say, with zero enthusiasm.

'It was,' she smiles. 'I am.'

'I'm very happy for you. What was the operation?'

'Sorry?' she asks, looking a little distracted, lost in marvelling at her own marvellousness.

I can't be bothered to repeat the question. I'm knackered, my girlfriend is an aggressive pisshead, and I stink of puke. I don't give a shit what idiot patient of hers woke up so splendidly.

'Nothing,' I reply.

'How about you?' she asks.

I should launch into a long description of the Lithuanian machete fight, but I simply don't have the energy.

'Nothing much,' I say.

'Oh, what time is it?' She checks her watch. 'I suppose that's about right, no? All you get in now are the night-shift workers?'

Sally is right. It's about this time of night that things are supposed to quieten down a bit, when even this city starts to run out of drunks to deposit on our doorstep. After about three a.m. the rhythm of A&E changes. Staff do eventually get a chance to eat something, put their feet up for five minutes, write some notes, have a chat with each other, or even with a patient. You can take a bit more time, a bit more care. There's more of an opportunity for a bit of bedside manner to come out, if you will. Also, if the hospital is near a large twenty-four-hour employer –

like, for example, the West Middlesex near Heathrow – then as Sally has just said, the night-shift workers start coming in. They don't have anything better to do. The TV is on, the place is warm, they may as well hang out here and get their bad foot seen to as soon as go home. But you know, if you had to pick a time to come down to your local A&E, then after three a.m. is one of the best. The queues are much shorter, and the doctors are a little less run off their feet.

'Jesus Christ!' says Ben, bursting through the doors of the common room like a man on at least four lines of coke, which I suspect he is by now. 'That was heavy, wasn't it?'

'One of the more random things I have come across,' I agree.

'You OK?' he asks. 'I saw the puke.'

'I'm not normally a puker,' I say, looking down at my shoes. I must do something about them.

'I'm sure,' he nods. 'But that brain . . .'

'What brain?' asks Sally. 'You didn't say anything about a brain.'

Ben tells Sally the whole machete story, and I have to say even she gags at the end, which makes me feel a little bit better about myself.

'That's amazing,' she says, finally. 'Are the police here?'

'Of course the police are here,' he replies. 'Two men cut to pieces and no one takes any interest? Although one copper is a little worse for wear.'

I leave Ben and Sally chatting each other up in the common room and slope off to deal with the vomit on my shoes. I sponge away and rinse them under the tap in the lavs, then use the hand blower to dry them off. They are a shitty old pair of

281

trainers, but I've used them more or less every day since I started here and they have coped quite well with all the piss, blood and puke thrown at them. Although having said that, looking at them now, I think I might get rid of them after this shift – a new job definitely requires a new pair of shoes, and these two are quite frankly a health hazard.

I walk back to the changing room and decide it is probably a good idea to send Emma a text message. I am going to kip down here for what's left of tonight, I think; I can crash for a few hours then crawl back home later. I don't think our relationship is much longer for this world, but if I text her and tell her I'm staying here that's one less thing to beat me over the head with.

I put my hand in my jeans pocket, and just as I pick up my phone it beeps. I've got an email message, something from Facebook. As I click on and open it, my jaw slowly slackens. It's from the girl who has just been here, Shannon. She walked out of here having had a miscarriage, and twenty minutes later she's asking me to be her Facebook friend. She has even written a message: 'Thanks for earlier, Doc. Mayb U and I cld have a drink sometime? It was nice to meet you.' Quite apart from the fact that doctors are not supposed to shag the patients, I am gobsmacked that she thinks it's even a possibility. I didn't meet her, I gave her a pelvic examination. We weren't introduced at a party. I didn't chat her up in a club. Or even buy her a drink in a pub. I put my hand up her fanny to make sure she wasn't going to haemorrhage. That is not the sort of thing you want to tell the grandchildren. I delete the message and turn off my phone. The girl needs help.

Back in the common room, Ben and Sally are still chatting.

Actually, judging by Sally's body language – legs crossed towards him, throwing her short nose back a lot as she laughs – Ben may well be in there. Well, it is end of term; they aren't going to see each other again. Not unless Sally develops a sudden need for a frozen forehead or fat puffy lips. I wouldn't be surprised if they found themselves a quiet consultation room before the hour is out.

Walking back towards A&E, I bump into Alex on his way to the toilets.

'Is it busy in there?' I ask.

'My Lithuanian is going into theatre in a few minutes,' he says. 'Sanjay is still trying to get someone up from the morgue to get rid of yours, as he's slightly freaking the drunks out.'

'OK.'

'But it's a bit quieter now, just three alcoholics, your corpse, my machete victim and an SHO battling to remove a six-month-old rotten tampon.'

'Oh.' I grimace. 'I've been there.'

'Haven't we all,' says Alex. 'Anyway, I've got to go and scrub in.'

'So, all right do you think for me to slope off for a sleep?'

'How long have you been on for?' he asks.

'Twenty hours or so.'

'Like the good old days,' he says. 'You should go and ask Sanjay, but I'm pretty sure you're fine. There are enough juniors in the place. Even if I do take one to assist me. That bloke with the VTMK gone yet?'

'Voice to melt knickers? Who, Ben?'

'That's the one.'

'He's in the common room chatting up Sally.'

'Sally the anaesthetist?'

'Yup.'

'That's not hard, everyone's had her,' he grins.

'Really? She doesn't look like she goes at all.'

'Like a barn door in the wind, apparently. Always the quiet ones.' And with that he walks off up the corridor.

Sanjay is on hold to the morgue, waiting for someone to come and collect the brainless corpse. I imagine the police will be wanting to have a good look at him and then he'll be sent off for autopsy, although cause of death is pretty damn obvious. The fainting copper seems to be back on his feet: he's asking two of the paramedics who brought the men in questions. One of his colleagues is sitting with the lacerated survivor, hoping, I imagine, to grab any snippet that might fall from his extremely drugged-up lips.

I am just about to tell Sanjay that I'm leaving for a kip when Kareem comes running in from reception. 'Jesus,' he says, looking from me to Sanjay and back again, 'can you come? I have never seen anything like it before.'

Sanjay drops the phone and I follow him into reception. Standing in the middle of the room, flanked by two terrified-looking mates, is a bloke with a face blown up like a balloon. As I get closer I can hear that the young man is wheezing like Darth Vader, gasping for air; his eyes are scarlet and he is shaking with shock. He suddenly falls to the ground, his legs buckling beneath him.

'Ryan! Ryan!' shouts one of his mates, crying and snotting and panicking and smacking his mate's hugely bloated face. 'Ryan!'

The other bloke just stands still and stares at the floor, rigid with fear. Someone in the waiting room screams. Another laughs nervously. But mostly everyone just stares in horror at the sight of Ryan coughing and gagging on the floor through his inflated head.

'He just went to be sick,' says the crying friend, his huge imploring eyes weeping at me, two columns of snot pouring down over the top of his mouth. 'He vomited and screamed and then this happened. We'd only been snorting Ritalin.'

'Quite a lot of Ritalin,' adds his mate.

'How many?' I ask.

'Grams and grams,' he replies.

'Your friend has vomited so hard that he has burst his oesophagus,' explains Sanjay, crouching down to inspect Ryan's neck. 'And his face is full of gas.'

'His oesophagus?' asks the crying boy.

'His throat,' says Sanjay. 'And we need to operate right away otherwise he will die.'

A ruptured, or burst, oesophagus is one of the charming complications more usually associated with alcoholics, or binge drinking. Either the oesophagus is weakened by persistent vomiting in the case of an alcoholic, and then ruptures, or the vomiting incident is so violent and traumatic (in the case of binge drinking) that the throat is torn open in one swift movement. It is obviously serious, extremely painful and life-threatening. Over 40 per cent of burst oesophaguses are alcohol-related, and 75 per cent of oesophagus cancer cases are also due to alcohol.

I have seen a few ruptured oesophaguses before, but this is

the first time it has been due to Ritalin, and this also happens to be one of the more violent ruptures I have seen. Ryan is not long for this world unless Sanjay and I act fast.

He is taken swiftly into A&E and pumped with morphine and antibiotics to prevent any infection from developing in the ripped tissue. He is then given a whole load of IV fluids to replace everything he's vomited. I offer to scrub in with Sanjay, but he insists that after twenty hours at the coalface I have given enough tonight and there is a very keen junior called Damon who is desperate to get some throat surgery under his belt as he has his eye on an ENT consultancy prize further down the line.

So I sit around for another ten minutes or so waiting, just to make sure that our Lithuanian is taken down to the morgue. I'm not sure if he has any family over here, but he has to be formally identified and bagged and tagged and reunited with his brain before the coroner can even begin to review his case.

The morgue is usually one of the more difficult departments of the hospital to find. Since we are in the business of saving lives, we perhaps don't like to announce our failures too much and therefore we don't usually stretch to particularly ostentatious signage. Run by the mortuary technicians who get between £15,000 and £18,000 a year, the morgue is a place of rest where relatives can go and say goodbye but it is also kept pristine so that if we need to, we can take samples from the corpses for pathological analysis. Or at least that's the idea.

There have been lots of scandals and incidents in the past where bodies were not properly stored in morgues, for example being kept on the floor. In one bizarre incident a

Muslim woman's body was covered in slices of bacon as a mark of disrespect. On other occasions corpses have had their pituitary glands harvested and sold on to make children's growth hormone. Even more extraordinarily, one mortician was caught having sex with a dead body – needless to say he was fired. But our lot always seem very straight and banal, or at least that's how they appear.

Eric has worked down in the morgue for years. At least I think that's his name. He is not the chattiest of souls and he doesn't wear a name badge. Conversation between us rarely moves beyond the words 'This the one?' and 'Paperwork?'

He arrives smelling strongly of disinfectant and cigarettes, grunts a few incomprehensibles at me and checks the corpse is dead. There are a few stories around about corpses coming back to life in the morgue, of technicians noticing them breathing just as they are about to put them on ice, so it's in their interest, as well as mine, to make sure the patient is definitely dead and most certainly no longer for this world.

He covers the Lithuanian with a sheet. 'Right then,' he sniffs, 'I'll be off.'

I point to the stretcher. 'Er, I think you may have left something behind,' I say.

'Oh,' he says as he nonchalantly clocks the brain and peels it off the stretcher and pops it under the sheet. Another wave of nausea hits me.

'You lot seem to have lost your touch,' he says suddenly as he sets the wheels in motion. 'We are having a busy night.'

4–5 a.m.

Dear God I am tired. It's only after you switch off and the adrenalin subsides that you realize quite how knackered you are. In the old days I would have been able to manage a double shift, no problem, and I would probably have taken Ian up on his offer of a nightcap, and stayed up until dawn remaining completely compos mentis, despite the brandies. But tonight I'm dragging my sorry arse into a bed.

As I leave A&E, Sandra is talking to Ritalin Ryan's friends, trying to calm them down and explain that their mate will be OK, despite busting his neck open. Their OCD-like itching and scratching and shifting about, as well as their highly emotive states, makes me think they are probably all high as well. Jason 'Meow Meow' Grove is fast asleep in his cubicle, waiting to be taken upstairs. The drunks on drips are also getting some shut-eye, they will probably have about an hour's grace before we start trying to get rid of them.

It's been a heavy old day. The hangover, the double shift, my drunk girlfriend, the endless presentations, combined with the bizarre emotional upheaval of leaving this place – it's no wonder I feel so tired.

I walk past Stacy as I shuffle up the corridor.

'Night,' she says.

'I'm off for a snooze,' I explain. 'I'm not sure how long for.'

'Night,' she says again. 'E15 is free if you want it.'

'Great, thanks.'

I make my way a little further along the corridor. The door to E12 is slightly ajar. It looks cosy and inviting and, more importantly, closer than E15. I push the door and turn on the light. I hear the scream before my eyes manage to focus properly. And when they do, I kind of wish they hadn't. Sally is bent over a transparent plastic emergency cot, her face pushed against the wall, her knickers and scrubs around her ankles. Ben has his underwear and scrubs around his knees and his buttocks are rippling and wobbling with enthusiasm as he takes Sally from behind. They stop for a second as they take in the fact that they have been busted. Sally looks at me, her eyes glazed, her cheeks flushed with lust.

'Carry on, Ben!' she barks, turning her head away from me and smacking a flat palm against the wall. 'I'm nearly there!'

Ben does what he is told, and I am the one left to mumble my excuses and leave.

It's normally a little smarter to lock the door, I think, as I head up the corridor. I'm not that shocked. When I was a student doctor you almost always slept with the person you were on call with. It was something to do, to pass the time, to numb the terrible boredom of it all. I think the uniforms helped a little: the old uniforms were always a little transparent, just to add that extra frisson, and plenty of nurses wore stockings, or hold-ups, which would also jolly up one's day. The nurses were definitely more up for it then too. But perhaps that was because I was younger and better-looking and dripping with excess testosterone; also, maybe it was down to the fact that there was little else to do in Sheffield. They used to do little tricks to get us out of our clothes. One of the old favourites was spraying our trousers with water from a syringe, and then offering to help us find something dry to slip into. And there are plenty of places to remove one's clothes in a hospital, no end of rooms and cubicles, and most of them have a bed, despite cutbacks and shortages, and most of them have a door that locks. So it really is only a question of finding two consenting adults.

I find E15 and lie straight down on the bed. I contemplate removing my shoes but I'm too shattered to be bothered even to do that. Lying down on the hard plastic-coated trolley/bed, I feel like I'm right back in my student days, and it brings a smile to my face. I loved those days. The bed in my digs was so shitty and uncomfortable you were almost chuffed to be able to sleep in the hospital. The digs themselves were dreadful, too. I think I spent the first half of the year thinking, I must get some curtains, and the other half not giving a shit. But we were never there, so what did it matter? And when I was, I was either pissed or asleep or both. It seemed pointless to bother making the eight-foot-by-ten-foot box room your own. Why would you? I think a few of the female doctors bought some cushions for their beds, but that was about the sum total of domesticity on campus.

As I lie there thinking of Julian and the ridiculous IV contraptions he rigged up so he wouldn't feel like shit the morning after the night before, there's a knock at my door. It is so gentle and I am so half asleep, I think I might have imagined it.

It happens again.

'Come in,' I say, sitting up on the bed. 'It's not locked.'

The door opens and Stacy is standing there, backlit by the strip light in the hall.

I am a little stunned and sleepy. 'Is everything OK?' I venture, not sure if I'm reading this increasingly interesting situation correctly.

'Um, I was wondering if you, um, would mind if I came in,' she says.

To say that this is every student doctor's fantasy is an understatement. It's almost as ubiquitous as the Hippocratic oath. I don't know of a single quack worth his stethoscope who has not fantasized about a nurse arriving in the middle of the night and helping him out in his hour of need. And thank the Lord above, here is Stacy to do just that.

'Well, um . . .' I find myself saying.

I know it's the end of term, as it were, and I know I will never see Stacy again, but I surprise myself. I don't think I can. Much as I would love to feel her soft warm body next to mine, much as I would love to forget the traumatic exhaustion of the last day, I don't think I can. I have a girlfriend at home, even if she does stink of cheap white wine and Bacardi breezers. I just don't think I can do it.

'Oh good,' she says, starting to take her tunic top off at the door. 'I just thought, what with it being your last night and everything, I might be quite—'

'Really, Stacy,' I hear myself saying, 'thank you, but no thank you.'

'Really?' She stops in her tracks. 'Are you sure? Just a quick—'

'No. Really. Very kind of you to offer and everything, but I do have a girlfriend.'

'Oh, right.' She rolls her eyes as she pulls her top down. 'If you're sure.'

'I'm sure.'

'See you later then,' she says as she turns and closes the door behind her.

I lie there, thinking about my day – about the people who have died, about June, about the men who were attacked by their machete-wielding mate – and then I think about what I have just turned down, about what might have been, and I feel a little daft. Stacy is lovely. Stacy is sexy. It might have been fun. I can only hope that Emma is worth it.

I finally fall asleep.

They always say that the hours between four and five a.m. are the dying hours in a hospital. The time when a patient is most likely to pop his clogs. There are many theories as to why this is so. The most scientific is that cortisol levels or adrenal levels in the body drop, making the person more likely suddenly to slip away. However, I think it's because it's the most popular time for the night-shift nurses to take a break. So they are either having a quick one with a consultant or dunking a biscuit into a cup of tea. Either way it's going to take them a little longer to hear an alarm bell.

I am falling into a deep sleep when there's a knock at my door.

'Come in, it's not locked.'

The door opens.

'Stacy?' I open my eyes and see one of the male nurses standing in the doorway. 'Oh!'

'You've got to come quickly,' he says, sounding a little panicked. 'They've found a body.'

'A body?' I say, stretching.

'Yeah, a dead body,' he adds, sounding like he's never seen a stiff before.

'So?'

'So we need you. All the other doctors are busy.'

'I'm not getting out of bed for a dead person,' I say.

'Sorry?' Now he sounds completely confused.

'The person is dead. What can I do to help now?' I yawn and lie back down. 'No doctor gets out of bed for a corpse.'

'Please,' he says, sounding completely pathetic.

For some unknown reason I find myself getting out of bed. The last time someone woke me up in the night I had a massive row with him. It was another junior doctor who wanted me to take the pacemaker out of a corpse, as he was my patient and he thought I might want the ash cash. It was very kind of him to offer and all that, but there's something totally abhorrent to me about delving around in a cold chest looking for a pacemaker. I told him I didn't want the £71 that badly and only to wake me again if there was a possibility of my doing some good. So why am I helping out this sod? Maybe because he said please and asked me politely.

Rubbing my eyes under the bright strip light, I follow him down the corridor, expecting him to lead me into A&E. Instead he takes me to the toilets.

'In there,' he says, turning away.

'Here?' I look at the sign. 'The Ladies?'

He nods.

Inside, the place smells of urine and stale perfume. There are three basins down one wall, two of which have dripping taps, and there's paper everywhere. The hand towel dispenser is empty, mainly because its contents are spewed all over the grey texture-tiled floor. The three toilet cubicles are open and there is toilet roll curling under the door of the two closest to the main door. Women, it appears, are just as messy as men when they go to the loo. What an appalling place to die, I think, as I walk towards the furthest cubicle. I push the door with my finger and it slowly creaks open. There, lying curled up on the floor in the foetal position, the heroin syringe still in her right hand, is Nadine, the prostitute I spoke to in the car park earlier. It is too sad really. Her mouth is open, her eyes are half shut, and her long dark curls are wet with the water from the leaking toilet. She is barefoot and still wearing her hospital gown, which gapes at the back. She is not wearing any underwear.

'She must be a patient,' says the nurse.

'Her name's Nadine,' I say. 'She's from Hepworth.'

'What's she doing down here?'

'Looking for a quiet place to shoot up?' I say.

'How long has she been here, do you think?'

'I'm not sure,' I say, feeling the body. 'She's still a tiny bit warm but rigor mortis is settling in her eyes. Two to three hours, maybe more. I saw her at about oneish, one thirty?'

'What shall we do?' he asks.

'Move the body back up to Hepworth and let them deal with it,' I say. 'They are quite used to dealing with bodies that have been dead for a few hours. The nurses there have been known to find bodies and put them back into bed to let the doctors deal with them in the morning.'

'Do you think so?' he asks.

'I don't see why not. She was one of theirs. I'll stay with her if you want and you can go up and get them.'

He scurries off up to the fourth floor while I stay with Nadine. Knowing her name and having seen her swaggering about the car park does make it a little worse, looking at her here with her mouth open and her buttocks hanging out. I pull her gown around her a little more neatly. There's no need for her to be completely degraded.

I turn around and catch a glimpse of myself in the mirror. I look terrible. My skin is waxy, my eyes are red and I have purple bags under my eyes. I could also do with a shave. I lean over a basin and splash some water on my face; I can see Nadine's dead body reflected in the mirror behind me. For some reason the reflection looks more creepy, like some alternative reality.

Before I have a chance to spook myself completely, the nurse returns with a few more nurses in tow. As old Hepworth hands, they treat Nadine's demise with complete nonchalance. How long ago was she found? When did I last see her alive? She had apparently been up on the ward causing havoc, pissing everyone off just a few hours ago. The sister had accused her of dealing on the ward; there had been shouting and swearing, which is probably why she had come down so many floors to take her hit. She had apparently been in and out of that ward for the best part of a year. They all kind of knew that she would come to a sticky end. There was no other outcome for her.

They make short work of Nadine, and within about five minutes her body has been packed up on a trolley and covered in a sheet and is being taken upstairs for the paperwork to begin. The nurse and I walk in silence back to A&E. He collars a cleaner on the way and asks him to close the toilets and hose down the area thoroughly before allowing the public back in the place.

Through the double doors, and the drunks on drips are beginning to stir. Sandra is bustling them awake, clearly thinking about making them a cup of tea and kicking them out soon. The last thing she wants is for the next shift to inherit a row of pissheads on their arrival. She likes to run a tight ship, and if she can possibly hand over an empty A&E in a couple of hours to Andrea, she will. It's a matter of pride.

It's all part of the new policy of getting patients out of hospital as quickly as we can. Early Discharge is one of the shiny new flagship policies. I've sat in endless meetings with endless physios and occupational therapists working out how to get rid of patients. It's one of those tricky things: you don't want to send a patient home so early that they can't cope on their own; equally they are a pain in the butt to have hanging around if all they have is a broken wrist. And we have to involve so many bloody people. Half the patients' houses don't cater for them and their broken leg, particularly if they are elderly or live on their own, and then we have to involve Social Services, or get home help organized, or arrange the loan of expensive equipment to help them get out of bed, wash, dress and go to the loo. By the time we've finished with all that jazz, we might just as well have kept them in for another week. The problem is that people don't have families any more; we have had to become their family. Only that's not really what the NHS was set up for. We are supposed to be here in a crisis. We are not supposed to take the place of your extended family.

And woe betide us if we kick them out and they come back! We are judged on our readmission rates, and they are rising. Something like 13 per cent of over-seventy-fives are readmitted within twenty-eight days of being dispatched back into the community, and that rate is rising, up 31 per cent in the last five years. The under-seventy-fives fare a little better, with an 8.6 per cent return within four weeks, but that's bound to get worse. Some local councils are so terrible at looking after their ex-patients that I've heard of pensioners asking that rather than run the gamut of their appalling aftercare, might there be a kindly doctor who is interested in participating in an assisted suicide?

But these boozing boys getting their vitamin B shots will be back by the end of the week, or at least within the next month. Some of them are homeless but a surprising number are not. They just live on their own and have no one else to talk to except a TV and a brandless bottle of vodka.

I shall miss this place, I think, looking around. It's a love/hate thing. Helping people at their most vulnerable – it's why almost all of us went into medicine in the first place. It's just all the other shit that goes with it that I find hard to deal with.

'Oh good,' says Sandra, a look of panic in her eyes. 'We've got an RTA arriving in five minutes and everyone's in theatre. You have to stay.'

5–6 a.m.

Sandra pages both Alex and Sanjay, who are in theatre repairing the sliced-up Lithuanian and the open-necked Ritalinhead, and there's no one else about expect for a couple of juniors who've been on drunk duty for the last few hours. Even Dr Death is scrubbed, in with some poor unfortunate sod with appendicitis. I send a nurse to hunt up and down the empty rooms on E corridor in the hope that I might find Ben still pleasuring the implacable Sally. But to no avail: it seems they've both disappeared off into the night.

So we have an RTA on its way with four young male casualties and three doctors on call to deal with it. And one of them, me, has been up for nearly twenty-four hours and the other two have six months' real-life training under their belt.

Stacy and Sandra grab the drunks and clear them out of the area. They walk them and wheel their IVs down to the CDU, to join the grannies and other alcoholics who have already been placed there. We then all stand by the double doors, waiting, braced.

I remember talking to a friend of mine who was working the day of the 7/7 London bombings and he said that not only was it carnage, it was also chaos. But somehow they managed to get through the first twenty-four hours. Mostly he remembers spending hour after hour with a nail brush in his hands, scrubbing flesh. It was his job to get all the tiny bits of shrapnel and grit out of the skin to prevent 'tattooing', where the flesh grows over the lumps and bumps in the skin and becomes pocked and pitted like a form of tribal art. He said that every-one coped with the initial shock and trauma and heavy workload rather well. It was a Thursday morning, and every-one worked flat out through Friday and over the weekend to help sort out the wounded. Then on the Monday his depart-ment was sent an email from those on high that said something like 'Well done for all your hard work, at least we know that our major incident plans do work, and we will be ready should there ever be a next time.' He said what they had completely failed to grasp was that all the patients, all the injured and wounded, were still there. They would be there for weeks, if not months, and they were sending out emails like the whole thing was over. All the beds were full and all the doctors were still flat out; they worked sixteen-hour days for the next four weeks at least. They worked weekends, too; no one took any breaks at all. It was exhausting, and some of the critically ill patients were in and out of operating theatres every other day. It wasn't an incident that they managed to get through in forty-eight hours, this was weeks and weeks of work.

Although this car crash is, of course, nowhere near that level, the ramifications will play out in this hospital for the next few weeks, if not months.

The double doors slam open and the paramedics come sprinting in, one after the other. The noise is awful – low-level screaming, moaning and writhing around in pain. The stench of burning flesh and petrol hits us too. Sandra's directing which resus each of them should go into and the nurses are rushing around with IV stands, heart monitors and bags of blood and fluids.

The first boy is completely covered in burns. His face is black, his hands are charred and his clothes hang in smouldering tatters off his body. Jesus Christ, I almost can't look. The paramedics have managed to put a line in his arm, which is a feat in itself. There's no way I would have found a vein.

'The driver,' says the medic, looking sweaty and exhausted. He's covered in black soot and stinks of petrol. 'Trapped behind the steering wheel,' he says, shaking his head. 'The car was on fire, we couldn't get him out. He's about seventy per cent burns. He's dead. Died in the ambulance.'

'Right,' I say, checking his chest and heart for breathing or any other sign of life. 'Yes, you're right. Over there.'

We push him to one side. We cannot help him now. We must focus on the ones we can help.

'Next,' I say, without wanting to sound heartless. 'Keep talking to me.'

The next two lads aren't in great shape either. One looks the wrong side of barbecued, his forearms so badly burned the flesh itself is practically cooked. The other looks like he's been through the windscreen and back, with lacerations to prove it. We secure their airways and pump them with as many painkillers and fluids as we can. The burns boy continues to scream the whole time; I think it's the shock as much as the pain. It sounds terrible. It is incredibly hard to handle something like this, and it's made worse by the fact that they are all under twenty. The paramedics don't know what happened. They think that drink and maybe drugs were involved. The lads seem to have driven off the road while going around a corner too quickly. But all they know for a fact is that the car rolled twice, blew up, and turned into a fireball. To be honest, it's touch and go for both these boys.

I'm more confident about the fourth casualty, who seems to have escaped the worst of the fire and much of the impact of the crash. His left arm is bust, half the road is still in his chest, one of his legs is twisted and he has an enormous welt across one shoulder, which may well be dislocated, but it looks like his seat belt saved him from the worst of it, and he's only slightly burned. I think he must have been in the front passenger seat, and managed to get out more easily.

We are working up these cases like clockwork. Stacy is running back and forth with more blood and fluids. We are trying to keep the burns boy from completely drying out, dressing his skin, trying to cool it and prevent the burns from going any deeper. But his blood pressure is rising, his heart is not coping with the shock, his system is completely overloaded. Suddenly the heart monitor attached to him goes from pumping nineteen to the dozen to that familiar monotone as he flatlines.

'Adrenalin!' I shout. 'Paddles!'

Stacy hands me the syringe, and I plunge the needle into the boy's IV bag. One of the SHOs, Aiden, charges the defibrillator.

'Clear!' he shouts, holding the paddles dramatically above his head, before leaning over and shocking the boy.

He barely moves.

Aiden steps back, waiting for his machine to charge, then shouts 'Clear!' again and shocks the boy a second time.

Again the boy doesn't move, and the heart monitor remains monotone.

We carry on this dance for another fifteen futile minutes. We'd normally call it earlier than that but he's young so no one wants to give up. But it's like some macabre hokey-cokey: we're all stepping in and out of a circle, all of us knowing exactly what is going to happen, but forced to go through the motions all the same. If only to be able to tell the boy's parents that everything was done to save him.

'I'm going to call it,' I say eventually, safe in the knowledge that no one will dissent. 'Time of death five thirty-three a.m.'

Over in the other cubicle they are fast losing the other lad. He damaged his sternum on the way through the windscreen and is bleeding slowly but surely into himself. The cuts on his arms, legs and face are too numerous and the trauma is too much for his young body to cope with. This has to be one of the worst car crashes I have ever had to attend to. Within minutes I hear once again the deathly monotone of a heart monitor; the high-pitched squeak as the SHO charges up his defibrillator; the shouts of 'Clear!' and 'Again!' coming thick and fast.

It's all over so quickly. Three young lives taken within the space of about thirty minutes – it feels like a huge body blow. The department is left reeling, punch-drunk from so much chaos, so much blood and burning, so many frantic attempts at resuscitation, so much death. And it all happened just as we were contemplating a sit-down, a cup of tea and a catch-up on a few notes, or maybe slapping a few backs goodnight and sloping off to bed. This job just seems to know when your guard is down and you're feeling in need of a little sleep. It's only then that it comes right back at you and hits you hard between the eyes.

All efforts are now concentrated on the sole survivor. He is moaning and mumbling, trying to speak through his oxygen mask. By the look of his injuries, after some extensive surgery, physio and rehabilitation he will probably survive this whole thing. Poor bastard. He'll be walking out of a place where his three best mates died to become the focus of everyone else's questions and everyone else's grief. I can't think of anything worse.

'How are they?' he manages to ask, his scared eyes looking from Stacy to me to Aiden.

'Let's not worry about them now,' says Stacy, putting a hand on his shoulder.

'They're dead, aren't they?' he mumbles through the plastic mask.

'Let's concentrate on you,' Stacy says.

'Angus is dead, isn't he?'

'Which one is Angus?' I ask.

'The driver,' he says, staring at me, willing me to say the opposite of what he knows I'm about to say.

'I'm sorry.'

Stacy shoots me a look like I'm not supposed to tell him. But I'm afraid I can't lie, and he has a right to know. They were all in that fireball together, and he must strongly suspect, otherwise he wouldn't have asked the question.

The young man squeaks. It's an odd sound. Like a baby working its way up to tears. He inhales a large gulp of oxygen and a tear runs down over his temple.

'And Mike?' he asks.

I bite the corner of my bottom lip and shake my head slightly.

The squeak is the same, but just that tiny bit louder. More tears flow down the side of his face and into his ears.

He can barely voice the last question he needs to ask: 'J-J-Jamie?'

'I am very sorry,' I say, taking hold of his heavily grazed hand.

He pulls it away from me and turns his head carefully to face the other way. His shoulders move slightly as he starts to sob.

He then turns back to look at me with bright-red eyes. 'All of them?'

I nod.

He inhales heavily again and looks at me furiously, like it was my fault. Then he lets out a low, awful wail. He tries to move his hands up to his face, but it proves too painful. The sobbing gets louder. He struggles in his bed, his legs and arms kicking. 'No-o-o–oo—ooo!' he shouts at the top of his voice before descending into a fit of coughing that brings two nurses running over.

'Will! Will!' says one of the nurses, pulling the sheets more tightly over him. 'You must calm down.'

'Leave me alone!' he shouts. 'Leave me alone,' he sobs. 'Leave me alone,' he whispers through his mask.

I back off. The boy is waiting to go up to X-ray himself; the last thing he needs is an audience for his grief.

I walk past the three corpses covered in sheets, waiting for their paperwork to be sorted and for Eric to come up and collect them. The first body is Angus, the driver of the car. His notes are clipped to a board at the bottom of his bed. I look a bit more closely at his chart; someone has written TTJ right at the very end: 'Transfer to Jesus'. It must be one of the juniors. I feel a surge of indignation course through my body. What student doctor dickhead wrote that? Maybe I'm tired and emotional, and call me old-fashioned, but I don't find three youngsters dying in a car crash a particularly rich vein to mine for comedy.

I am on the verge of shouting at a few people when Alex arrives fresh from stitching his Lithuanian back together.

'What's happened? I got your page. Jesus . . .' he says, looking around the place. 'It looks like a car crash in here.'

'It was, it is,' I say. 'Three dead, one of them DOA.' I rub my face.

'I'm sorry, mate,' he says. 'The nurses don't pass on the pages when you're in theatre. Any survivors?'

'A young man, cubicle four, Will,' I say. 'Late teens, broken arm, dislocated shoulder, potentially fractured pelvis, and I'm sure there are a few more things going on. He's about to go up for X-ray. He also needs half the road scrubbed out of his chest.'

'God.' He sniffs, looking over at the three dead boys lined up in a row. 'It looks bad.'

'It was,' I nod.

'You should take a minute,' he says. 'Go outside. Have a cigarette.'

'I might actually go home,' I say. 'You've got the new lot in an hour or so.'

'I know,' he says, raising his eyebrows. 'That's something to look forward to.'

Now that Alex has mentioned it, I realize I am desperate for a cigarette and some solitude, so I go outside and light up. The sun is just up; the sky is a pale blue and the clouds are pink with a hint of purple. It looks like it might be a nice day. I pull out a cigarette and realize I must have left my lighter some-where. I look around the car park and see a bald-headed bloke parking his car. I wait for him to get out of the car before going over.

'Excuse me,' I say, 'do you have a light?'

'I'm sorry?' he says, looking a little puzzled.

'A light?' I say, waving my cigarette by way of a serving suggestion. I know it's early in the morning.

'Oh, right,' he says, tapping down his pockets. He then holds his head in his hands.

'Are you OK, sir?' I ask.

'I've got one in the car,' he says.

He turns around and I immediately perform a double-take. As the man bends down to look in the passenger-seat glovebox he gives me a perfect view of a huge hole in the back of his head. I lean forward to take a closer look. Not only has a large part of his scalp disappeared, so has the skull. I can see right the way through to his brain.

'Excuse me,' I say. 'I don't want to be rude, but you appear to have a hole in your head.'

'Oh, yes,' he says, 'that. That's why I'm here. I'm feeling a little dizzy.'

6–7 a.m.

I'm not sure how long I would go around with a hole so deep and gaping in my head that you can practically see the inner workings of my brain, but this old boy, Martin, has been quietly going about his business with his brain open to the elements for a whole goddamn year!

'Doesn't it hurt?' I ask, as I escort him towards A&E.

He shakes his head. Apparently not.

'How did it happen?'

He explains that he had a small patch of skin cancer on his scalp and his wife, being a homeopathic sort of a woman, had decided that doctors were shit and what he needed was some sort of red wort tincture, which is from some North American weed. She has been applying the stuff every day to the patch on his head. The only thing is, skin cancer can be quite sensitive to what you put on it, and this stuff seems to have inflamed the cancer instead of calming it down. In fact, the thing has been so goddamn inflamed it has managed to bore a hole right into his head. The hole is actually big enough for me to put my fist in. No wonder the bloke feels a bit dizzy. There's trepanning to let a little bit of fresh air into the brain to help with the blue-sky thinking, and then there's creating your own sunshine roof.

'How do you shower or have a bath?' I ask, my body shivering at the thought of Badedas on the brain.

'Oh,' he says, looking at me like I'm asking the weirdest question. 'I wear a showercap.'

'Right,' I say. 'I suppose it does the trick.'

I take Martin straight through and sit him down in a cubicle. Within five minutes all the doctors on call have come in just to have a look. Sanjay can't believe it.

'He's been going around like that for a year?' he checks.

'It seems so,' I say.

'He looks in remarkably good condition. That's a big plastics job if ever I saw one. They're going to have to replace the skull and grow him some new skin.'

'It's going to take a while.'

'I know a bloke who can fill almost anything,' he says. 'Nice chap. He loves a challenge. I'll give him a call.'

'Now?'

'Men like him don't need sleep,' says Sanjay. 'Sleep is for the weak, remember?'

'And in the meantime?'

'In the meantime . . .' He pauses. 'Fluids.'

'Of course,' I say. 'How could I forget?'

Martin is hooked up to an IV just to keep him busy. He's

been offered painkillers but he's turned them down. So I leave him leafing through a six-week-old copy of *Now* magazine. Sanjay's on the phone outside, calling round, trying to track down his superior plastics chap. I can hear the words 'huge hole in his head' and 'yeah' over and over.

I walk back through the department. The three car-crash corpses have thankfully disappeared, but Will, the survivor, is still here. He must be waiting for his X-ray. I poke my head in through the curtains. His eyes are closed – the drugs have kicked in now. He looks a little more comfortable despite his smashed-up face and broken body. I am about to leave when he opens his eyes.

'Oh, sorry to disturb you,' I begin. 'I was just checking you were OK. It shouldn't be long now for the X-ray. I'll go and see what's holding them up.'

I know he can hear but he doesn't react. There is no flicker of recognition, no acknowledgement that I am trying to help. He just stares at me over his oxygen mask. The look in his glazed eyes makes my blood run a little cold. He blinks slowly, then looks away.

'OK then,' I add, 'I'll go and look.'

Before I can get anywhere near the computer, a very large, very vocal woman comes screaming into A&E, accompanied by a panic-stricken man. 'It's coming, and it's coming right now!' she yells, stopping to grab hold of a trolley. She lets out a positively primordial roar that brings the whole department to a halt. Blood and water whoosh on to the floor.

Alex drops his clipboard and comes running over. 'Here, in here,' he says, skidding slightly in the puddle on the plastic floor. 'Let me help you.' He grabs hold of the woman and tries to push her towards a cubicle and a bed.

He's a braver man than I.

'You!' bellows the woman, turning to look at him with her scarlet cheeks and bloodshot eyes. 'Just fuck off!'

'OK, fuck off, absolutely,' says Alex, realizing his mistake. It is not terribly advisable to try to shift a woman during a full-blown contraction.

The husband/partner just looks around in blind panic, trying to work out what to do, and where to go. His eyes lock on to mine. Oh shit, I think, here we go.

'Here,' I say, moving towards a cubicle and pulling back the curtain, 'this one's free.' I approach the pregnant woman with caution. Women in labour are so strong and determined, they have been known to fell a consultant with one swift well-placed punch. 'In your own time,' I say to her. 'When you are ready.'

The contraction subsides and she begins to list slowly in the direction of the cubicle. Alex stands there, feeling a little bit useless.

'Um, I'll phone Maternity,' he says.

'You do that!' yells the woman, leaning so heavily on my shoulder I think my legs are going to buckle.

'Here we are,' I say, patting the bed.

'Oh my God!' shouts the woman, again.

Her knuckles turn white as she grabs my shoulders. Her grip is hard and deep, her long red nails dig into my back. I want to join her as she screams out in pain. There's another whoosh as more water and blood pour over the floor.

'I'm really sorry,' she announces suddenly to me and the husband/partner, 'I need to do a poo.'

'Oh my God, man,' says the husband/partner.

'Don't push,' I say. 'Hold on.'

'Nooooooo!' she yells. 'It's coming!'

'Jesus Christ!' declares the husband/partner.

'Don't push!' I shout, getting down on my knees and putting my head up her huge floating skirt.

'I have got to poo!' she screams.

'Man, get your head out of there!' yells the husband/partner.

'Oh shiiiiiiit!' the woman wails, almost squatting on top of my head.

'OK, I can see the baby,' I say. 'Push!'

'The baby?' asks the husband/partner.

'Yes!' shouts the woman. 'What the fuck do you think I'm doing here?'

The husband/partner's reply is, fortunately for him, interrupted by the arrival of a midwife.

'What in God's name are you doing?' she asks me, her short arms crossed over her large chest. It's like she's telling off a three-year-old. 'Get yourself out from under there, will you? Are you all right, love?' This question she directs to the woman. 'Why don't you sit yourself up here and let's have a look at you. Oh my goodness, I can see Baby's head. You've done so well, just a few more pushes and Baby's out. My name's Monica. And you are?'

'Lorraine!'

'OK then, Lorraine, just do exactly what I tell you to do and you and Baby will be fine. When I say push, you push, and when I say stop, you stop. OK?'

'OK!'

Monica sits on the bed then looks at me and the husband/partner in a manner that implies a certain amount of irritation at the fact that we are still here. We both read the look and retreat, at speed.

While the two of us wait for Lorraine to bring a new life into the world, aided and abetted by the firm forearms of Monica, A&E prepares itself for a changeover. The backlog is cleared, Will is finally taken up for an X-ray, and the juniors are next door handing out sugary tea and sandwiches to the alkies, telling them in no uncertain terms that they don't want to see their ugly mugs again. I go in to help them, and among the tramps, the down-on-their-lucks and the other pissed-and-fell-overs, I spot my businessman, the one who pissed himself. He's sitting in the corner, rather forlornly eating a roll. Spending a night in stinking damp trousers curled up next to an incontinent granny can't have done his hangover much good. The man's mouth looks so miserably dry; he can barely get enough saliva together to get the doughball down his gullet. One thing's for sure, and I'd be prepared to bet money on it: he won't be back in here for a while. It's a pity half the other drunks who spend their nights here don't feel equally chastised.

Over in the far corner, closest to the bin, I spot a woman lying horizontal on the red plastic chairs. She doesn't appear to be moving. In her early twenties, wearing a pink-striped T-shirt, a short black skirt and cheap red heels, she is very obviously a prostitute. I look a little more closely and notice she is covered in track marks. Her arms and wrists are pricked pink and raw. I check her pulse. She's still breathing, so I haul her up to a sitting position. She mumbles something before slumping forward. She's high as a kite, whacked out on heroin. Beside her is a small black leather handbag, which is lying open. I pick it up and look inside. Maybe someone knows who she is? Maybe someone should come and get her? What is she doing here in the first place? The contents of her bag are covered in a brown dusting of heroin. It's everywhere, all over the condoms, her keys, her empty purse, the photo of what I presume is her daughter and a small box of Kellogg's Coco Pops. It is all too pathetic.

I look at her, passed out on the chair, her long dark hair stuck to the side of her face, her dark brown lipstick smeared, one of her hoop earrings missing, and I think, what should I do? She's alive, she's not about to die. I could phone Social Services, get them involved. Or I could just walk away. It is the end of my shift. The end of my time here. I have been on the go for twenty-four hours. And they'd only make me stay another two hours while we filled out some more forms, signed a few things, and she'd be back out on the streets by the end of the day. So I walk across to the tea trolley, make a cup of very hot, very sweet tea, and put it at her feet. I can only hope she wakes up before it gets cold.

Back in A&E, I bump into Monica, who is dumping her white plastic apron in the bin.

'A boy!' she says, looking a little short of breath. 'She sure as hell did make a noise.'

'That's nice,' I say. 'The dad must be thrilled.'

'That's two sons in one week for him,' she says. 'He

was with another woman giving birth in here at the weekend.'

'Which one is his wife?'

'Maybe neither of them,' she says, with a smile.

The next time I look at the clock it's ten minutes to seven, not long now before all the doctors arrive box-fresh from medical school. As each of the juniors, like Aiden, who have spent the last six months or so cutting their teeth in A&E walk up to say goodbye to Sandra, I can see the panic begin to rise in her eyes. The idea of turning up tomorrow to a department entirely staffed by new recruits is clearly beginning to freak her out. She's smiling and nodding her goodbyes while nervously sorting through things, making neat piles of sterilized swab kits and moving the piles of cardboard bedpans to one side.

'Excited about today?' I ask, preparing to say goodbye myself.

'Nothing I like better than a whole load of arrogant incompetents who can't even find a vein,' she says.

'I know, but we all need to learn some time,' I say, wondering how open the arms of the consultants in Acute Medicine will be in St Patrick's down the road.

'Yes, of course we have to learn,' she agrees. 'Just maybe not all at once.'

'There is that.'

'Worst day to be ill in the whole year.'

'I know.'

'It's that lot out there I feel sorry for,' she adds, pointing her bony finger at the waiting room.

'Well, bye then,' I say, shaking her leathery hand. 'See you soon.'

I look around for one last time. I'm going to miss this place. The people. The stories. The unexpected.

'Oh, I'm glad I caught you!' says a nurse running towards me. I recognize her. 'Thank you for helping us out earlier with the woman.' She nods towards the toilets that are still closed for cleaning. 'We all just wanted to give you these. To say thank you.' She hands me a large box of Terry's All Gold.

I look at them. They are dented in one corner. Then I look across at the office where I last saw the A&E box. It's no longer there.

'Are you pinching the staff chocolates?' asks Sandra, coming over to investigate.

'No,' says the nurse. 'They're a present from Hepworth Ward.'

'Really?' says Sandra, leaning in. 'Those were our chocolates yesterday.'

'They were?' asks the nurse.

'I'm all for regifting,' says Sandra, 'but perhaps not back to the same place?'

The nurse looks mortified. Two pink patches appear on her cheeks.

'The thought was there,' I say, smiling at her before handing the box back to Sandra. 'These chocolates have been here since 1986. I don't think they should ever leave.'

Sandra possessively puts the box back in the office and I take one last look at the place.

'Have you signed out of the computer?' asks Sandra, coming back out of the office.

'Oh, right,' I say.

'And leave your password,' she adds.

I am soon poised over the computer, thinking I might leave the new boys a note saying 'Don't take any shit from Sandra, be nice to Stacy, and Margaret is a bit of a goer.' I could also advise them not to get involved with the drunks or the junkies, and let the abuse and the swearing wash off their duck's backs. I want to tell them to listen to the patients – to what they don't say as much as what they do. And don't, if they know what's good for them, ever admit anyone with back pain. The consultants won't thank you, the hospital won't thank you, and you'll never get rid of the bastard. But I don't. Instead I pick up a pen and find a piece of paper. I am ready. I am off. Oh, what the hell is my password?

Imogen Edwards-Jones is the bestselling author of *Hotel Babylon*, *Air Babylon*, *Fashion Babylon*, *Beach Babylon*, *Pop Babylon* and *Wedding Babylon*, as well as novels such as *My Canapé Hell* and *Shagpile*. She lives in west London with her husband and their two young children.